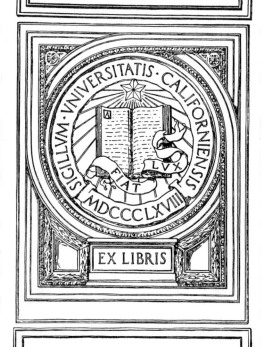

RADIATION THERAPY
AND THANATOLOGY

RADIATION THERAPY AND THANATOLOGY

Edited by

RICHARD J. TORPIE

LEONARD M. LIEGNER

CHU H. CHANG

AUSTIN H. KUTSCHER

KENNETH L. MOSSMAN

and

KENNETH LUK

With the Editorial Assistance of

Lillian G. Kutscher

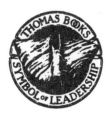

CHARLES C THOMAS • PUBLISHER

Springfield • Illinois • U.S.A.

Published and Distributed Throughout the World by
CHARLES C THOMAS • PUBLISHER
2600 South First Street
Springfield, Illinois 62717

© *1984 by* CHARLES C THOMAS • PUBLISHER
ISBN 0-398-04885-1
Library of Congress Catalog Card Number: 83-4989

With THOMAS BOOKS *careful attention is given to all details of manufacturing
and design. It is the Publisher's desire to present books that are satisfactory as to
their physical qualities and artistic possibilities and appropriate for their
particular use.* THOMAS BOOKS *will be true to those laws of quality that
assure a good name and good will.*

Library of Congress Cataloging in Publication Data
Main entry under title:
Radiation therapy and thanatology.

Bibliography: p.
Includes index.
1. Cancer—Radiotherapy—Psychological aspects. 2. Cancer—Patients—
Family relationships. 3. Terminal care. I. Torpie, Richard J. [DNLM: 1. Neo-
plasms—Radiotherapy. 2. Death. 3. Ethics, Medical. QZ 269 R1282]
RC271.R3R332   1984   616.99'40642   83-4989
ISBN 0-398-04885-1

Printed in the United States of America
PS-R-3

CONTRIBUTORS

RICHARD J. TORPIE, M.D., *Associate Professor of Radiation Therapy, Hahnemann University Medical College and Hospital, Philadelphia, Pennsylvania; Director, Radiation Oncology, St. Luke's Hospital, Bethlehem, Pennsylvania*

LEONARD M. LIEGNER, M.D., *Assoicate Clinical Professor of Radiology, College of Physicians and Surgeons, Columbia University, New York, New York*

CHU HUAI CHANG, M.D., *Professor of Radiology, College of Physicians and Surgeons, Columbia University, New York, New York*

AUSTIN H. KUTSCHER, D.D.S., *President, The Foundation of Thanatology; Professor of Dentistry (in Psychiatry), Department of Psychiatry, College of Physicians and Surgeons, Columbia University; Professor of Dentistry (in Psychiatry), School of Dental and Oral Surgery, Columbia University, New York, New York*

KENNETH L. MOSSMAN, Ph.D., *Associate Professor and Director, Graduate Program in Radiation Science, Department of Radiation Medicine, Vincent T. Lombardi Cancer Research Center, Georgetown University Medical Center, Washington, D.C.*

KENNETH H. LUK, M.D., *Associate Professor of Radiation Oncology, University of Washington, Seattle, Washington*

RUSHDY ABADIR, M.D., *Professor and Chief, Department of Radiation Oncology, University of Missouri-Columbia Hospital and Clinics, Columbia, Missouri*

ISAMETTIN M. ARAL, M.D., *Chief, Therapeutic Radiology, Long Island Jewish-Hillside Medical Center, New Hyde Park, New*

v

York; Professor of Radiology, State University of New York at Stony Brook, New York

THEODORA ARNOLD, C.R.T., Administrator, Department of Radiation Therapy, Southern California Permanente Medical Group, Los Angeles, California

SUCHA O. ASBELL, M.D., Clinical Associate Professor, Department of Radiology, Temple University School of Medicine, Philadelphia, Pennsylvania; Division of Radiation Therapy, Temple University School of Medicine, Philadelphia, Pennsylvania

HARRY L. BERMAN, M.D., Head Emeritus, Division of Radiation Oncology, Sinai Hospital; Adjunct Associate Professor of Radiation Oncology, University of Maryland School of Medicine, Baltimore, Maryland

PHILIPPE B. BRICOUT, M.D., Assistant Professor of Radiology and Assistant Director, Department of Radiation Medicine, Boston University School of Medicine, Boston, Massachusetts

ARTHUR C. CARR, Ph.D., Professor of Psychology in Psychiatry, New York Hospital—Cornell Medical Center (Westchester Division), White Plains, New York

JOSEPH R. CASTRO, M.D., Professor, Radiation Oncology, University of California, San Francisco, California

PATRICIA CHAMBERS, M.B.A., R.T.T., Administrator, Department of Radiology, The Presbyterian Hospital in the City of New York, New York

NINA H. DIAMOND, M.S.S., Department of Radiation Therapy and Nuclear Medicine, Thomas Jefferson University Hospital, Philadelphia, Pennsylvania

EDWARD H. GILBERT, M.D., Former Program Director for Radiation Therapy, Radiotherapy Development Branch, Division of Cancer Treatment, National Cancer Institute, Bethesda, Maryland; Director, Peter A. Lake Memorial Radiation Center, Rancho Mirage, California

JOHN W. HARRIS, Ph.D., M.D., Associate Professor of Radiation Oncology, University of California, San Francisco, California

JEAN HATTEM, R.N., Behavioral Medicine Department, Southern California Permanente Medical Group, Los Angeles, California

A. R. KAGAN, M.D., Chief, Department of Radiation Therapy, Southern California Permanente Medical Group, Los Angeles, California

LILLIAN G. KUTSCHER, *Publications Editor, The Foundation of Thanatology, New York, New York*

P. LEVITT, Ph.D., *Professor, Department of English, University of Colorado, Boulder, Colorado*

TRISH LITTMAN, *Doctoral Candidate in Sociology, University of Pennsylvania, Philadelphia, Pennsylvania*

JAMES MCKENZIE, M.S.W., *Department of Social Services, Boston University Medical Center, Boston, Massachusetts*

NORMAN L. MAGES, M.D., *Associate Clinical Professor in Psychiatry, University of California, San Francisco, California*

Y. MARUYAMA, M.D., *Professor and Chairman, Department of Radiation Medicine, University of Kentucky A. B. Chandler Medical Center, Lexington, Kentucky*

MOHAMMED MOHIUDDIN, M.D., *Profesor of Radiation Therapy and Nuclear Medicine, Medical College of Thomas Jefferson University, Philadelphia, Pennsylvania*

RABBI STEVEN A. MOSS, *Coordinator, Jewish Chaplaincy Services, Memorial Sloan-Kettering Cancer Center, New York, New York; Spiritual Leader, B'nai Israel Reform Temple, Oakdale, New York*

ROBERT H. SAGERMAN, M.D., *Professor and Director, Radiation Therapy Division, State University of New York Upstate Medical Center, Syracuse, New York*

EGILDE SERAVALLA, Ph.D., *Research Associate, Department of Anesthesiology, Beth Israel Hospital and Medical Center, New York, New York*

WILLIAM J. SOBOTOR, B.A., R.T., *Clinical Coordinator for Education, Radiation Therapy Program, State University of New York Upstate Medical Center, College of Health Related Professions, Syracuse, New York*

JEROME J. SPUNBERG, M.D., *Clinical Assistant Professor, Temple University School of Medicine; Attending Physician, Division of Radiation Therapy, Albert Einstein Medical Center, Philadelphia, Pennsylvania*

S. A. TAUSEND, Ph.D., *Assistant Professor, Department of Sociology and Behavioral Sciences, University of Kentucky, Lexington, Kentucky*

ARNOLD WALD, M.D., *Assistant Clinical Professor of Radiotherapy, Albert Einstein College of Medicine of Yeshiva*

*University, Bronx, New York; Attending Radiotherapist, New
Rochelle Hospital Medical Center; Medical Director, Comprehensive Cancer Care Team, New Rochelle Radiology Associates; Private Practice, Rye, New York*

RICHARD WHITTINGTON, **M.D.**, *Department of Radiation Therapy
and Nuclear Medicine, Thomas Jefferson University Hospital,
Philadelphia, Pennsylvania*

PREFACE

This book is dedicated to the memory of Dr. Bernard Schoenberg, one of the cofounders of The Foundation of Thanatology and a major influence in the development of the area of caregiving known as thanatology. Although it seems so very appropriate that this book be introduced in such a fashion—particularly because Bernie's own medical care required the use of radiation therapy—any of my efforts to think of a memorial or a eulogy to him appear inappropriate and inadequate when referring to a man who seems to be still with us in our presence in spirit and in memories that do not dim. Consequently, most of what follows was written while he was still alive and will, I hope, put into context the philosophy of caregiving on which this book is based.

I first met Bernie when he was a resident in psychiatry at the New York State Psychiatric Institute in 1957. His intelligence, dedication, and humanity were apparent then, and in recommending him as a psychiatric resident to the Foundations Fund in 1958, I had occasion to write:

> In summary, I feel that . . . Dr. Schoenberg is eminently qualified for your support. I do not feel this trust in him would be misplaced but that it would be an investment in one who would go on to contribute immeasurably to mental health. . . .

Eighteen years later, in 1976, I had occasion to state my subsequent experience and evaluation of one who had become in those years a dear and valued friend and collaborator:

> As an example of Dr. Schoenberg's ability to organize, supervise, and inspire the execution of a multicontributor research design, I would

point to the project which ultimately reached publication as "An Investigation of Criteria for Brief Psychotherapy of Neurodermatitis." Using 20 psychiatric residents whom he personally supervised in their treatment of the patients, Dr. Schoenberg brought together service, training, and research goals in a way that, to my knowledge, has never again been duplicated in our department. This study was meant to serve as a model for an approach to the treatment of specific disorders with specific treatment methods—an approach that was not generally utilized at that time. Great reservation and suspicion existed about precipitous symptom removal that would presumably result in regression and the development of new symptoms. We have subsequently seen the development of many other specific approaches to specific symptoms, but the study was indeed one of the first demonstrated approaches and has, I believe, implications for psychiatry which have not yet today been fully realized.

Continuing this evaluation, I wrote the following:

An example of Dr. Schoenberg's innovative skills as applied to the area of teaching was that model established for the teaching of psychosocial aspects of patient care to students of the health professions. Utilizing a multidisciplinary faculty, he succeeded in integrating behavioral science concepts in all spheres of the nursing school curriculum. The model was later applied to other student groups, such as with the dental school. In the Foreword to the volume *Teaching Psychosocial Aspects of Patient Care,* of which Schoenberg was the senior contributor and editor, Dr. H. Houston Merritt wrote, "The model of teaching described in this volume reflects the feeling that a function of the University is to assume leadership for research in providing quality medical care for large numbers of patients."

Thanatology is another area in which Dr. Schoenberg's leadership and foresight have had profound influence. When loss and grief first became a possible focus of interest in terms of founding an organization that would play a role in education and research, death was indeed a taboo topic. Within a few years, Columbia-Presbyterian Medical Center became internationally known for its contribution to the field of Thanatology. Its publications, symposia, research, and educational programs have had wide impact. The book, *Loss and Grief: Psychological Management in Medical Practice* (with Schoenberg as senior author and editor), is considered the first medical textbook in the area. The climate has now changed—it is hard to keep up with all the books appearing on death or dying—but this major shift, along with its impact on the education of medical students, was brought about primarily through support of Dr. Schoenberg to Dr. Kutscher [and his colleagues in thanatology].

As further evidence of his human and humane interests in health care problems, a more current project might serve as a final example. Aware of the ethical dilemmas and the value conflicts that are arising on almost a daily basis that relate to health care in our rapidly changing society, Dr. Schoenberg has fostered the development of a Journal that is to provide a forum for the discussion of the crucial issues, "Man and Medicine, The Journal of Values and Ethics in Health Care." With the recognition that health care stands at the junction of numerous and diverse disciplines, as many relevant points of view as possible are to be brought to bear: those arts and sciences traditionally defined as comprising medicine; new professional specialties including those being developed in the allied health fields; the natural and social sciences and the "humanistic disciplines" as well. It is this broad kind of focus Dr. Schoenberg believes should be brought to bear on health care problems.

My 1976 statement closed with this paragraph:

> I would not close this presentation without some comment on Dr. Schoenberg's abilities as a clinician. I believe he is a psychoanalyst in the finest sense of the word. He is empathic, insightful, patient, understanding of the complexity and depth of human feelings yet not so preoccupied in "listening with the third ear" that he fails to hear with his two ears. He is the psychiatrist I would want for a relative or loved one, and that, I suppose, is about the highest praise one can give any physician.

All this is now past. Life does go on, and we must remind ourselves that mourning is not the only way to respect and do honor to a dead loved one, nor should it be used to rationalize passivity. The Foundation of Thanatology originated from a personal loss that motivated vigorous and creative action. No, grieving is not the only way to hold a loved one close. Our real challenge is to emulate those qualities which so endeared to us those who are the object of our grief. We must be the carriers of their immortality, whatever other kind might also exist. In relation to Bernard Schoenberg, this task seems herculean, but with the help of such people as have contributed to this book, I think it can be done.

ARTHUR C. CARR

ACKNOWLEDGMENT

The focus of the discipline of thanatology is on the art of enhancing humanitarian caregiving for patients who are critically, chronically, or terminally ill, with equal concern exhibited for the well-being of their family members. From a base in thanatology, interdisciplinary professionals are dedicated to promoting vastly improved psychosocial and medical care for these patients and assistance for their families. Proposed is a philosophy of caregiving that reinforces alternative ways of supporting positive qualities in the lives of those who are critically ill, life-threatened, or dying and that introduces methods of intervention on behalf of the emotional support of their family members and bereaved survivors.

The editors wish to acknowledge the support and encouragement of The Foundation of Thanatology in the preparation of this volume. All royalties from the sale of this book are assigned to The Foundation of Thanatology, a tax-exempt, not-for-profit, public, scientific, and educational foundation.

CONTENTS

Contents

RADIATION THERAPY
AND THANATOLOGY

Section I

THE PATIENT
AND RADIATION THERAPY—
ART VERSUS SCIENCE

Chapter 1

RIGHTS OF PATIENTS
A Thanatologic Perspective on Cancer Caregiving
RICHARD J. TORPIE

I t is important to note that cancer is an age-related disease, with increasing incidence with increasing age. By 1985, the first group from the post-World War II baby boom will turn forty. At that point, over 50 percent of the population will be over forty years of age, and, therefore, more prone to cancer. Simultaneously, that portion of this population will remain healthier and, for a longer period of time, will be more available to cancer. This disease incidence is directing the medical community to take a prospective look at some of the problems that will arise in the next twenty years.

How are health professionals preparing themselves for this inevitable future? Facing them, medically, financially, and psychologically will be a crisis in cancer care, and this must affect thanatologists who deal with the practical end of the concept of a patient's emotional care.

Cancer is most often used as a model for psychosocial caregiving. However, it must be considered in terms of a generational disease, that is, a disease toward which the attitudes are widespread, rooted with various subgroups of patients' personal, familial experience, both favorable and unfavorable. Because of the lack of psychosocial support, these attitudes may be completely devastating when cancer is confronted in the family system. A crisis exists when perhaps as many as 5 percent of patients now presenting themselves for radiation therapy refuse to initiate or do not complete treatment for reasons based on their beliefs and the myths that have been handed down within the family or other social network.

Susan Sontag (1978) has stated that "as long as a particular disease is treated as an evil, an invincible predator, not just as a disease, most people with cancer will indeed be demoralized by learning what disease they have. The solution, then, is to hardly stop telling cancer patients the truth, but to rectify the conception of their disease and demythize it."

Several years ago, a group of Philadelphians from various disciplines met to talk about what prevents us from accomplishing the numerous modes of psychosocial support for the cancer patient. The questions asked were, What is wrong? What tends to keep things wrong? The list included the primary reality of *institutionalization,* which basically consists of those policies and traditions in hospitals which foster dehumanization and depersonalization. One of the first things that happens to a patient passing through the hospital admissions office is the affixing of a band with a number on his wrist and the removal of certain valuable or personal articles from his possession. The patient ends up in a strange, white, sacklike gown not looking much like himself anymore. These policies and traditions may produce priorities that, especially for the cancer patient, can provide a milieu of poor quality of care, often reflected in the absence of a caring presence, the lack of time for giving care, and the loss of empathy.

We also see a *lack of true informed consent.* Duff and Hollingshead (1968) pointed out that in many situations, the cancer patient about to undergo surgery, radiation therapy, or any other therapeutic procedure is often denied an accurate representation of what the treatment may do to him. The urgency of the decision to do something is often forced on the patient. When a patient is told that a mandibulectomy or a laryngectomy will be performed, he often does not realize what this means and may undergo a procedure that, although lifesaving or cancer arresting, will be totally devastating for his life-style.

In some cases physicians *hide behind their terminology.* There is also *chronic compartmentalization of medical specialties,* where often the cancer patient, and more often the sicker terminal patient with cancer, falls between the cracks of responsibility and is left without channels of communication, finding himself to be the only expert about what is happening to him.

In other cases our death-denying society has not been educated with regard to dying. Only limited skills exist for dealing with the emotions that surround cancer. Many of the leading medical school institutions use a "Band-aid" approach that barely touches the needs of patients. Profit-making organizations or the profit motive within the medical system and the relative callousness of the third party providers do not reflect the need for emotional support of patients in the hospital. Yet, anything that provides for such emotional support and serves to make the patient feel better, whether mentally, physically, or emotionally, often leads to fewer hospitalizations and better care outside the hospital. In the long run, it is profitable to support the patient emotionally.

Many professionals are unable to cope subjectively with cancer. If a physician cannot empathetically relate to patients with chronic wasting illnesses, he should not accept responsibility for their care. Rigid traditionalism is used as a barrier, male chauvinistic fears of emotionalism exist, and the unfair stereotyping of patients with terminal disease remains. There are disease prejudices in nursing as well. One example was the case of a fine elderly lady who, when the author was on his rounds, showed him a container of sour milk on her tray. When he brought it to the nursing station, someone remarked, "It's all right—she has cancer." Subtle things emerge, but the view that a person can be expendable is clear.

Societal, hierarchical, and community structures within a hospital system impede dealing with new issues. The rights of both patients and families to participate in matters of concern to them are denied. Most importantly, with repeated hospitalizations, continuity of care for the patient is lost. Rehabilitative input to patients, especially those who have cancer, is lost. People seem to use the word *rehabilitation* only for those patients who are totally salvageable, or curable, and not for those who are terminal. Yet Holland and Frei (1973) define rehabilitation as "helping the patient to adjust to altered body image as well as to the limitations placed on him by his disease and treatment, whether successful or not. Proper management entails a commitment to achieving optimal patient function and satisfaction from life, during and after therapeutic procedures, for as long as the patient lives." With this goal, enhanced by psychosocial support, optimal patient well-being can be achieved without considering total curability.

The author came from a rather protected environment of a medical school where, because of large staff diversity, students had limited exposure to the terminally ill. Often, in a training position, responsibility could be shrugged off or diminished, and innumerable consultations could be had. One thing in this environment made an impression, however—the loss of continuity of care.

During the author's residency, his most distinguished mentors formed a trio of very concerned and caring oncologists with extensive clinical expertise in caring for the cancer patient. Even they were basically unsupported by the department of psychiatry or the department of social work. There was no integration of effort.

From this hospital, the author went to practice in a hospital serving a small community. In 1973, there were 300 new cases of cancer in this institution; in 1980, there were 950. Suddenly, there was a realization that this meant trouble. The medical oncologists, some surgeons, and a very basic social services department approached the state American Cancer Society for help. The hospital received funding to start up a psychosocial cancer care group to be directed by a doctoral candidate in social work. She designed an excellent program with medical staff cooperation and the help of pastoral care. Joining the team were a former visiting nurse, a social service worker with family therapy training, and a psychiatric social worker with an interest in cancer patients. Within this community of some 250,000 people were innumerable individuals with education and resources who had never been utilized for community cancer activities but who became available to the staff once this program was started. For patients, there was no end of the need to tap continually the resources of volunteers and others. What was needed and accomplished was a maximization of total community support and resources for the support of the cancer patient.

Most of this effort was basically an emotional and social support system. Whenever possible, a member of the cancer care team was with the patient within days of the time of diagnosis. Team members were made available to the patient and the family at the time of revelation of recurrent disease, often more devastating to the patient than the initial diagnosis. Booklets in English and Spanish provided information of all types for the patient. Other resources in the community provided a base for family emotional support. Also created was a system of advocacy, the kind of advocacy in which people could come back for a second or more adequate explanation after the physician or nurse, hiding behind language, had given a lengthy explanation that nobody would admit not understanding. The staff also inaugurated cancer support and education groups within the community.

The author was surprised when he gave his first lecture to a community group to find patients he had treated four, five, and six years earlier. They had remained frozen in the community, frozen with fear of recurrence, frozen with inability to live a full life although most probably cured of their disease. What good is it when medical staff do the right thing and provide for cure or prolongation of life in worthwhile ways if the patient who is the object of all this cannot do the living? With this new support, the staff found themselves able to communicate informations with confidence and without inducing paralyzing fear, especially in situations involving recurrence and incurability. In the past, the patient with the highest likelihood of metastatic disease—the patient with lung cancer or breast cancer— was not given accurate information of what might be anticipated from this disease. If a patient with oat-cell cancer of the lung has had radiotherapy and some chemotherapy and there has been repeated regression of a primary tumor, is it right that this patient should not realize that there could be problems with spinal cord epidural metastatic disease or other problems that are highly likely but that can be minimized in early stages? The author and his colleagues have been educating patients in this regard. As a result, when there is evidence of metastasis, the problem is caught early and not when it has become totally catastrophic. This allows for continued control and worthwhile quality of life for the patient.

The thrust of these efforts has helped to demythicize cancer. There is a spontaneous continuity of hospice or terminal care programs started with a home-care basis, not as a free standing hospice facility. Interestingly enough, there has been a tremendous referral and education-seeking movement from other small hospitals regionally. The program has also tried to delineate the solutions to the problems facing community hospitals in maximizing good cancer care. The author's hospital was selected to participate as one of the new generation of community hospital oncology programs by the National Cancer Institute.

Having faced critical situations and presented possible solutions, the medical community should now able to talk about what is wrong and how things might be, what the ultimate idealism might be, and what an individual would want if he were a cancer patient. In these visions, the patient should be an equal and full member of the health care team. Supporting family relationships while the patient is hospitalized is of paramount importance. Medical services should be available, unencumbered by administrative bureaucracy that magnifies health care costs and the problems related to health care.

For example, in some situations the patient is in a private room for the first three hospitalizations, a semiprivate room for the next four hospitalizations, and in a ward for the last two hospitalizations. A simple adjustment in a computer can guarantee that a patient, once treated for an illness, will, on repeated admissions to the hospital, come to a floor with nursing staff and others who are at least familiar with his care. At times it seems that hospitals might borrow comfort systems and architectural ideas from hotels and resorts. In the typical semiprivate room, there may be a senile or disoriented patient with sheets over her head, her nightgown on the floor, with everybody walking by her open door despite the fact that nurses left her in a presentable state only two minutes before. By turning the angle of the room 90 degrees and adding small screens, one could give this patient privacy, even with the door left open.

Patients should be better educated about their bodies, to which end the author and his colleagues obtained closed circuit television cassettes that try to explain cancer and radiation therapy clearly.

There must be an end to the apparent elitism in medicine that separates the physician from the nurse from the social worker. How many physicians know many nurses' names on a floor where they have worked together for years? The anonymity that exists does not benefit the patient with cancer. This patient, too, has the right to the information on his chart, a right to information on his x-rays, a right to privacy—including the privacy of a locked door if necessary. There is a need for patients to be able to let the staff know if everything is not going all right, and advocates should be empowered to be involved in the patient's care.

A patient should have the right to decide whether or not there will be an autopsy. People dedicated to the cure or the control of their own disease like nothing better than to make this final gesture, but it is often denied them because of sentimental distortion by a relative who may not have been closely involved. There should be equity and not just efficiency in dealing with patients of all types and of all ages. Open communication is essential. Without communication and recognition that patients with terminal disease are people of value, medical care will never achieve the true milieu that will allow for better patient care. In their dealing with cancer, physicians—even those who are radiation oncologists—must utilize their own defenses in a continuing way to meet the confrontation of patient care every day. They must leave behind something of themselves when they deal with patients, or they are not empathizing with them directly and fairly. They must have support available to them also.

Hypotheses often talk about hope in an ambiguous and abstract way. It then often becomes a fantasy, and a fantasy that often becomes distorted. Fantasy and false hopes should be reduced and dissipated if life is to become meaningful. If true support is not available, the patient will be shortchanged by inappropriate care.

When the author first went into radiation oncology, colleagues would ask how he could stand it. The public readily distinguishes the diagnostic radiologist from the therapeutic radiologist and often with great uneasiness. Radiation therapists also seem to share a certain isolation from the remainder of the medical community. If anything, they are the most misunderstood group in medicine. Often in other specialists' minds, anything related to or unrelated to cancer can be blamed on radiation. This unfounded impression denies patients appropriate support from referring physicians. So long as this misperception exists, there will be a block to humanizing patient care.

The radiation oncologists have responsibility as well to let themselves be known within the hospital environment and within the scientific community. They must let it be known that they can offer patients true hope, not a vague carrot on a stick, but a well thoughtout promise for a good quality of life, no matter what the clinical situation might be. Avery Weisman (1972) gave a fine definition of hope when he wrote, "Hope is having confidence in the desirability of our survival. It arises from a desirable self-image, a healthy self-esteem, and belief in our ability to assert a degree of influence on the world surrounding us." A nineteen-year-old Vietnam veteran, who had leukemic infiltration of the esophagus before he died, lay in his room surrounded by books and promises of the future life that he could no longer live. When he was asked what his definition of hope was, he said, "Hope is the ability to fulfill oneself as one is." This truly encompasses the rights of patients with terminal illness.

Too often medical staff walk away from the darkened room where a terminal patient lies weakened, not cleaned, crowded by medical apparatus, and perhaps carelessly dressed and groomed without the things about him that mark him as a person who has lived, loved, and is still part of life. This person is the one who the most needs the finest care and attention. Sometimes the radiation oncologist is called in consultation as a desperate last measure, an inappropriate gesture. The author entered the room of a comatose man who had stomach cancer that had metastasized to brain and bone. He was obviously experiencing his last day of life, and the medical oncologist and the internist could not explain the reality of what was happening to the family. In a few minutes of the evening, the author found himself awkwardly making eye contact with a family whom he had never met before: a loving daughter, the man's wife who was still dreaming of a miracle, and his sister from California who was newly arrived and shocked with the scene. Unfortunately, no one had asked for the cancer care group to intervene. The author found himself in the presence of this family in this limited, vital, important time with a man who was beyond all thought of therapy. He had lived his life; he was still breathing but deeply comatose, and, in effect, comfortable. The wife's denial was obvious, so the author had her sit next to him, and as he held her hand he said, "I can't help this man—I can't perform miracles. He wouldn't let me perform miracles because he would just have to die all over again." Slowly, as reality set in, everyone wept because all had somehow been able to share in the common humanity that surrounds people.

George Bernard Shaw said that life is a state of disease that we are all at, one way or the other, somewhere. We must be able to cope with this on every level. Medical personnel must be able to be not only physicians, technicians, or nurses but feeling people who are able to accept other resources being made available from thanatologists, social workers, anthropologists, and all others ready to give part of themselves. Then they will be able to deal with cancer on the realistic level as a total disease affecting the total person, the total family, and the total community.

REFERENCES

Duff, R.S. and A.H. Hollingshead. 1968. *Sickness and Society*. New York: Harper and Row, pp. 365-85.

Holland, J.F. and E. Frei. 1973. *Cancer Medicine*. Philadelphia: Lea and Febiger, p. 498.

Sontag, S. 1978. *Illness as a Metaphor*. New York: Farrar, Strauss and Giroux, p. 7.

Weisman, A.D. 1972. *On Dying and Denying—A Psychiatric Study of Terminality*. New York: Behavioral Publications, Inc. p. 20.

Chapter 2

MEDICINE AND THE DYING
Different Attitudes through Time
EGILDE SERAVALLI

In the past, when science was not so advanced as it now seems to be and modern techniques were just starting to find their way into medicine, death was not regarded as the end of a biologic process. Rather, it was considered a problem that neither science nor logic could resolve. As a consequence, when physicians and medical staff became aware of the limitations of their knowledge and the uselessness of medical devices to delay the natural course of a disease, they ceased their efforts and respectfully allowed the patient to die.

From the Middle Ages until the middle of the nineteenth century, medicine was considered a humanistic science. The majority of illnesses, often leading to disastrous ends, were regarded as having been predetermined by fate. The family doctor (with no way to control these illnesses) cloaked his medical impotence with a bedside manner, or a more truly humane approach to the declining patient and the members of his family. During this extended historical period, suffering was considered as a necessary premise for a dignified and noble acceptable death. It was borne with deep resignation because it was considered a means to rescue man from the pettiness of his finite limitations and to raise him toward a consciousness of universal values. Suffering was valued as a device for giving the individual time to become aware of death's imminence, and medical practice was influenced more by philosophic questions concerning the nature

14

of human existence than by the indiscriminate use of the equipment then available.

From the middle of the nineteenth century until yesterday, technological knowledge interceded to divide up the patient into anatomical segments and fragmented the doctors' understanding of him as whole being. As a result, the work of this phase has tended to make the human body and its pathologic states the object of ever-increasing intellectual curiosity. During this period, it became more difficult to speak of medical art and more appropriate to speak of medical science. Having put its trust in the power of reason, medical technology developed sophisticated devices that, when used in a terminal illness, seemed to lengthen the sometimes long road to death. Instead of prolonging meaningful living, physicians sought to delay the end of life, even though they recognized that death was imminent and inevitable.

The apparent success of technology has distracted physicians from considering medicine as something more than an agglomeration of hypothesis, facts, and techniques that need experimental proof. Basically, medicine is a humanistic discipline, since it concerns itself with the human being as an entity unto itself. The differences between the earlier practice of medical art and its present practice so influenced by technology must be emphasized because the passage from one to the other has brought about a radical change in the relationships between doctor and patient, doctor and illness, and patient and illness.

The medical generations trained according to a technological culture see the patient as a living organism to be studied, examined, and sometimes experimented on in specific scrutiny of its biological responses. It is almost as if medical science were in competition with death to see which of them will carry the prey. The patient—a subject with sensations and thoughts—is set aside or, rather, transformed into an object. This figurative reference to man as an object of dispute recalls an early nineteenth century visual representation entitled "Life and Death." In it, the prey is fought over by a magnificent female figure and a pouncing terrifying hag on the other.

As we approach the end of the twentieth century, physicians are beginning to acknowledge their primary function as medical caregivers, that is, not to act as intermediaries in the final struggle between life and death but to act as mediators in helping human beings to accept the final transmutation. The medical community is becoming aware that technological values, important as they are for progress, can never be totally severed from humanistic values.

Although most physicians still believe that as long as physiologic life has a chance it is their responsibility to support this chance, a few doctors are tempering their efforts as signs of impending death become evident. These few have realized that intellectual curiosity alone leads to fragmentation of scientific knowledge. They have rediscovered man in his totality, a being of body and spirit.

This approach restores the medical presence to the bedside as a sensitive and compassionate human figure and not a powerful and manipulating force. The medical community seems to realize that the very success of its achievements has intruded into the right of patients to direct decisions that belong to them and only to them.

Doctors of medicine wish to understand death in order to give it meaning within the context of human existence. They recognize that many individuals, denied an awareness of imminent death, will never be able to end life in harmony with the self. These doctors wish to restore to their patients the possibility of making decisions concerning themselves. They seem willing to accept once again the patients' integrity as free human beings, not objects or means, but subjects and ends in the final struggle between life and death.

For the present, then, the roles are reversed. The dying become the teacher, and the doctor, the student. The doctor, a respectful and even a timid student, is faced by a new teacher who imparts knowledge at the very moment he himself acquires it. Simultaneously, the doctor makes a series of discoveries that, if communicated, lead to enlarged human awareness. The value of this human awareness transcends the value of any technological discovery.

Those close to the dying recognize that they know, see, and feel truths that may be verified experimentally only at the particular moment in which these realities are experienced. Until that moment, no scientific proof will permit man to discover and hear these truths.

According to Ziegler (1978)—

> The process of dying can be identified neither with life nor with disease. It is rather the chronological terminal phase of existence and of the epiphenomenal consciousness. . . . It has nothing to do with normal biophysiologic life nor with its pathologic states. . . . The process of dying implies a change in personal identity, and it is a succession of events of different orders. The death process slowly changes perceptions, attitudes, and even the sense of connection with physical reality. At the end of the process, the dying person may be quite different from what he was at the beginning. (P. 145)

This need to integrate medicine with the humanistic disciplines as well as with the scientific is not a backsliding process. On the contrary, it is a maturation process that represents the highest expression of spiritual and intellectual development. From the immediate past, we have scientific methods that may be used to transform technicoscientific knowledge into a means by which human beings may achieve, not the conquest of death, but an understanding of the significance of death in relation to their place in the universe. This would not deny modern science or its achievements but rather curb its application when it interferes with the freedom of man. In this way, modern science can be an instrument for the preservation of genuine human values, a goal of any human spirit.

REFERENCES

Ziegler, J. 1978. *The Living and Death*. Rome: Mondadori (translated by the author).

Chapter 3

RADIOTHERAPY FROM THE PATIENT'S VIEWPOINT

PHILLIPPE B. BRICOUT AND JAMES MCKENZIE

INTRODUCTION

Although much has been written about the patient's attitudes toward cancer, his anxiety about anesthesia, his grief over surgical mutilation, his sense of loss and fear of death, only an extremely limited medical literature covers the subject of the psychosocial effects of radiation therapy. Radiation therapy as a therapeutic modality can be misunderstood by the general public and the patient, as well as by the physicians themselves (Peck and Boland, 1977; Peck, 1972). This chapter does not propose to be an exhaustive catalog of patients' reactions to and problems generated by this therapeutic modality. Rather, it offers a qualitative outline of the most salient points as perceived through interviews of 100 radiation therapy patients carried out by a social worker (J. McKenzie) and presents, not a systematized and quantified analysis of these, but a distillation of the entire experience of the patients interviewed.

THE TREATMENT

Radiation therapy consists of a protracted course of four- to five-times-weekly treatments, which are often stretched over a period of five to eight weeks. The treatments are not painful; in fact, there is no feeling to them at all. The patient lies in an immobile position on a stretcher while the radiotherapy machine is positioned meticulously every day. Carrying out this procedure may take five to ten minutes on a difficult case. After this, the technician leaves the room, a heavy lead-shielded door is closed, and the machine is turned on. The technician remains in contact with the patient either through a small leaded-glass window or a closed circuit TV system with an intercom. The treatment lasts an average of one and a half to five minutes. Prior to the initiation of treatment, all of these procedural details are explained to the patient. The lack of sensation or pain as an accompaniment of radiation therapy is especially stressed.

THE PATIENT'S ATTITUDE TOWARD TREATMENT

The patient's first reaction to radiation therapy, after all the explanatory details have been given and all the reassurances emphasized, is, "This is going to be easy." After all, there are no knives, no needles, no anesthesia, no nauseating chemotherapeutics. How can something that is painless and that involves only a few minutes a day be such a problem? (Of course, there are other fears and worries that the authors will address later.) However, as the course of treatment is followed, such side effects as loss of appetite, nausea, and fatigue, as well as local reactions within the radiated field, increase in magnitude. In contradistinction to the surgical treatment, where a frightening and traumatic event, the surgery itself, takes place as the first definitive step toward curing and is followed by a period of convalescence with a gradual increase in the patient's feeling of well-being, the radiation treatment, seemingly nonthreatening, becomes a process of attrition in which a well patient gradually becomes sick, tired, and depressed over a period of several weeks. It can become a wearing, debilitating process, demanding all of the patient's energy for just getting back and forth to the treatment center and surviving the side effects.

THE PATIENT'S SUPPORT SYSTEM

Close family and friends who represent the patient's immediate support system during the illness do not understand the difficul-

ties of radiation therapy. Surgery and pain are readily compre-
hended, and the sympathetic visits to the patient's bedside,
flowers, and words of encouragement are liberally given. When
radiotherapy starts, sympathy is not that readily available.
Everyone knows that the treatment does not hurt, but the
debilitating nature of the side effects is difficult for anyone who is
not actually undergoing the treatment to understand. In the
beginning, a well-meaning family will encourage the patient,
telling him that it will be easy. This, of course, reinforces the
patient's attitude through the first, or benign, phase of radiotherapy. As the second, or debilitating, phase is ushered in, the
family's understanding lags. This, for the patient, tends to close
the door on further recrimination. The idea expressed or implied
is, "I can't understand what there is to complain about," and
perhaps, "You are pampering yourself."

There are also logistical problems for getting the patient back
and forth to daily treatment sessions. Many patients are unable to
drive themselves, and this imposes on family or relatives who have
other obligations besides a fairly long commitment to daily taxi
service. This role reversal tends to make the patient feel helpless
and gives him the feeling that he is being a burden to others. The
taxi service spreads the burden of radiotherapy from the patient to
the family, who may become weary of the entire process. This
depletion of the patient's emotional environment is often
exacerbated by the fact that radiotherapy for some patients is the
second or third line of treatment. Indeed, by this time, the patient
is often emotionally on his own.

FEARS

For the patient undergoing radiotherapy, many fears are
present (Peck and Boland, 1977; Rotman et al., 1977; Mitchell and
Glicksman, 1977). Immediate fears are generally related to the
claustrophobic aspects of the treatment. The patient must be
closed in the treatment room, which has been sealed with
radiation-proof doors, and remain alone with the machine.
Contact with the technician through the intercom system, for
some people, increases the sense of aloneness, and being separated
from the outside by the heavy doors instills claustrophobic

reactions of varying degrees. In one of the authors' patients, this was so pronounced as to necessitate the technician's talking to her continuously through the intercom.

Another fear is that the machine will drop or fall on the patient lying helplessly on the treatment couch, crushing him to death or perhaps only injuring him. Peck and Boland (1977) have reported similar concerns. Although such incidents have, in fact, happened, they are fortunately rare occurrences. However, the constant recurrence of this fear suggests that it is not associated with the accident itself but more probably with the extreme proximity of the machine to the patient's body, especially when shadow trays bearing blocks or other devices are attached to it, further reducing the free space between the patient and the machine's projections.

Machine malfunction and the fear of being given an excessive amount of radiation, permanently damaging the tissues, are also sources of concern. Patients are very sensitive to the amount of time that they are given treatment, and even minor adjustments of the time created by either the nature of the machine or adjustments following the recalculation by the physics staff will be perceived and will be questioned: "Why am I receiving a different time than I did yesterday?" The malposition of fields is also an important concern for the patient, and he will notice very minor discrepancies in field setup and will comment anxiously about this. In addition to the previously mentioned fears, the patients also harbor the traditional concerns about radiation, namely, skin burns, hair loss, nausea, and vomiting as well as sterility and future potential cancer induction (Peck and Boland, 1977; Rotman et al., 1977; Mitchell and Glicksman, 1977). These fears reflect popular knowledge about A-bomb victims. Although some of them are justified, others are not. Indeed, the patient has probably been told by the radiation oncologist or the radiotherapy nurse prior to the initiation of treatment that the radiation will kill good cells as well as bad cells as they attempt to describe the possible hazards of radiotherapy.

Peck and Boland (1977) have described strong feelings occurring in patients during their radiotherapy treatments. While some patients may have positive feelings, such as that the malignancy is being destroyed, others have negative thoughts about the possible deleterious effects of radiation on their normal tissue. Some workers have attempted to potentiate the positive feelings by mental exercises focusing the patient's concentration on the destruction of malignant cells by irradiation (Simonton et al., 1980).

PALLIATIVE AND CURATIVE RADIOTHERAPY

One of the misconceptions held by the general population and, indeed, also, unfortunately, by many physicians is that radiation therapy is not a curative technique. This tends to transmit the impression that patients referred for primary radiotherapeutic management are, therefore, "incurable" (Peck and Boland, 1977). Radiotherapy can be used in many ways, either primarily with curative intent or as an adjuvant therapy, pre or postoperatively. Whatever the situation, the patient is rarely ever transferred to the radiotherapy department with an adequate concept of the reasons for the referral. It is difficult for the patient to understand that radiation may be as curative as surgery. Often questions are asked, such as, "What happens to the tumor when it is destroyed by the rays?" "Where does it go?" Perhaps the image of cutting it out has such powerful impact on the imagination that it is impossible to think of surgery as being anything but curative. It remains difficult to convince the patient and family that a course of curative radiotherapy will do the job and that this does not represent a second line of treatment for a malignancy that has become too far advanced for definitive management (Rotman et al., 1977). The family will politely listen to explanations in the presence of the patient and then return afterwards to ask, "Now you can tell me the real truth, how long does he/she have to live?"

Palliative radiotherapy presents a different problem. Here the goal is admittedly limited to alleviating a distressing symptom such as pain, bleeding, obstruction, and the like. The disease is already disseminated, and a fatal outcome is sealed. The family understands all of this; however, the patient, who by this time is living his life from day to day, will have a generally positive response to palliative radiotherapy. For him, palliation is cure. Yesterday's distressing symptoms have yielded to the benevolent radiation. Cassileth et al. (1980) report that fully one-third of patients receiving palliative therapy as compared to one-half of those who were treated radically thought that radiation therapy might cure their disease.

THE PATIENT'S RELATIONSHIP TO THE MACHINE

As in other forms of medical treatment involving machinery, a very special relationship often arises between the patient and the radiotherapy machine. Some patients may see the machine as not merely a tool of treatment, which is what it is, but almost as a god that has to be pleased and placated to reward him with cure. This god exacts tribute in the form of radiation sickness, nausea, and multiple other side effects and complications. The rather strict daily schedule of radiation treatments is seen as an inexorable framework within which little bargaining can be done. Indeed, the patient may bargain to have the time of the day changed, the time of the treatment changed, but he may not have the treatment cancelled for a major reason. Technologists represent the human element with which the patient generally has a very positive relationship (Peck and Boland, 1977; Mitchell and Glicksman, 1977). They will go to great lengths to make the patient less fearful and more comfortable, talking to the patient, adding a pillow here, a wedge cushion there. However, there are some things the technologist cannot do, and in that sense this professional is a servant of the machine. For example, a patient who is rendered phobic by machine movement may want to bargain that the machine be positioned first and that he be allowed to creep onto the table and position himself under the beam. The technologist must say that this, unfortunately, is impossible to do because of the limitations of the machine; the machine is then seen as inexorable, allowing for little or no bargaining.

Sometimes the radiation oncologist may be seen more as the "high priest" of the machine than its master. If, for example, a particular dose of 5,000 rads has been planned for the patient, written on the chart, and further enshrined by the calculations of the physics department, and if at a given time the radiotherapist decides to stop short of this goal because of patient reaction, he will have great difficulty in explaining to the patient why this modification will not jeopardize the chance for cure. The patient, having received 4,000 rads instead of 5,000 rads, will be hard pressed not to think that he has been shortchanged and thus will have a diminished survival because the norm has not been filled and the rigidly planned schedule has not been carried out. Patients will react negatively if the treatment is prolonged ("My case must be bad since I need all these treatments.") or if the treatment is curtailed ("Are they quitting on me because I am incurable?"). In addition, there is a definite anxiety that occurs during rest periods—the fear that the tumor will grow during the period of discontinued treatment.

COMMUNICATION

The patient who arrives at the radiotherapy department with many misconceptions as a result of his own lack of knowledge and, perhaps, erroneous information from his referring physician ("You'll only need a few treatments.") is given a lot of information during the first interview by the radiation oncologist. There is evidence that he retains very little of this and only infrequently asks questions. The information must be repeated at another session.

While the beneficial effect of information on alleviating the patient's anxiety has been reported upon by some (Cassileth et al., 1980), others have stressed the basic lack of communication between radiation oncologist and patient (Rotman et al, 1977; Mitchell and Glicksman, 1977). Patients appear to be reluctant to seek information from the radiation oncologist. It has been suggested that mental health professionals could represent a third party to whom the patient could turn for emotional support.

In the authors' experience, the patient is also more likely to seek information or reassurance from either a social worker, a radiation technologist, or other patients. The generally good rapport between radiation technologist and patient has been stressed earlier. The authors' experience would tend to contradict that of Mitchell and Glicksman (1977), who state that patients tend to talk to technologists only about trivialities, and would seem to agree with Peck and Boland (1977), who indicate that patients relate better to technologists than to radiation nurses and better to nurses than to radiation oncologists. This is probably because they meet on a daily basis with the technologist and thereby have a chance to build up a relationship over the period of the treatment. They see the nurse less frequently and their radiation oncologists usually only once a week.

Other factors are also involved. Rotman et al. (1977) state that often the physician has no time or desire to listen to and communicate with his patient. The authors believe that this is only partially true. The have attempted as a general policy to have enough time for an unhurried first interview, but this does not appear to have altered the communication difficulty. There is considerable anxiety associated with the questions that arise in the patient's mind, and this anxiety probably prevents him from questioning the person who really can offer pertinent information. The patient may be so dependent upon his physician that he does not wish to disturb or possibly anger him and thereby jeopardize his treatment. Finally, denial is often the mechanism of defense in cancer, which will interfere with the adequate transmission of information. For all these reasons, the patient is paradoxically the most ready to talk to the person who can least respond to his questions. In order to be an effective communicator, one must release only as much information as the patient actually desires to know. This requires considerable sensitivity and experience.

CONCLUSION

The authors have offered a brief outline of some 100 patients' concepts of and feelings associated with a course of radiotherapy treatments. Many of the fears and concerns are genuine; others are definitely irrational or magical in nature. The careful student of human nature would be wise not to scoff at this, since when one's life is threatened, more primitive forms of thinking are called into existence. Behavior that seems irrational becomes totally understandable in this context. There is great need for further studies in this subject to achieve clarification of some of the conflicting findings as well as quantification of the frequency of some of the reactions described.

REFERENCES

Cassileth, B.R., D. Volckmar, and R.L. Goodman. 1980. The Effect of Experience on Radiation Therapy Patients' Desire for Information. *International Journal of Radiation Biology and Physics, 6:*493-96.

Gottschalk, L.A., R. Kunkel, and T. Wohl. 1969. Total and Half-body Irradiation Effect on Cognitive and Emotional Processes. *Archives of General Psychiatry, 21:*574-580.

Mitchell, G.W. and A.S. Glicksman. 1977. Cancer Patients: Knowledge and Attitudes. *Cancer, 40:*61-66.

Peck, A. 1972. Emotional Reactions to Having Cancer. *American Journal of Roentgenology, 114:*591-99.

Peck, A. and J. Boland. 1977. Emotional Reactions to Radiation Treatment. *Cancer, 40:*180-84.

Rotman, M., L. Rogow, G. DeLeon, and N. Heskel. 1977. Supportive Therapy in Radiation Oncology. *Cancer, 39:*744-50.

Simonton, C. et al. 1980. *Getting Well Again.* New York: Bantam.

Chapter 4

THERAPEUTIC TECHNIQUES TO CONTROL THE INNER ENVIRONMENT OF THE RADIOTHERAPY PATIENT

STEVEN A. MOSS

This is an account of a morning in a hospital's radiotherapy center.

The outpatients sat on one side of the wall in the waiting area. Some were dressed in their street clothes; others wore the loosely fitted blue gowns that showed they were ready for their treatments. Few people spoke with anyone else. Many stared solemnly ahead as they waited their turn. The inpatients were placed in direct sight of the doors that housed the machines. They could see the control booths in operation. Through the hustle and bustle of the technicians, they would watch those patients scheduled before them go in for treatment and then come out again. Most of these inpatients seemed to be exhausted. They sat in wheelchairs or lay on stretchers, either with their eyes closed or with their eyes wide open staring at the ceiling. As I looked at these patients I wondered what they thought or felt concerning all they saw and experienced.

I walked to the control booth that was stationed beside the visible treatment rooms that housed cobalt machines as well as a betatron and a megatron. The scene was like a page from a science fiction novel.

The machines were large and towered over the average-sized person. On the front of each room's door there was a sign that read CAUTION: HIGH RADIATION AREA. The control booth was entirely computerized, and it allowed the technician to manipulate

27

the machine and to communicate with the patient without entering the room.

I watched as they wheeled a patient into a room. I turned to the remote TV set, which showed the patient being positioned on the table. The only audible conversation was between the technician and patient and related to the patient's position on the table. After the technician left the room, the door automatically closed. The timer was set, and a red button marked "fire" was pushed. What was the patient thinking about as she lay alone under that huge machine?

After this visit to the radiotherapy treatment center, I began to wonder about the emotional state of the patient under the machine. I shortly discovered that there were no books devoted entirely to this aspect of radiotherapy. Only small sections in the textbooks for doctors, nurses, and technicians addressed the emotional aspects of the treatment. One author wrote (Watson, 1974),

> It is evident that patients in radiation therapy have as primary problems fear, depression, apprehension, and discouragement. Many of the patients will be suffering discomfort or, in some cases, very severe pain. Their introduction to the massive equipment used in many of the treatments may cause them anxiety. The fact that they are all alone in the room during treatment will tend to emphasize their concern. The problems in patient care of the radiation therapy patients are well known to most technologists but not necessarily easily solved.

Another author listed twenty-four possible questions that might be on the mind of the patient before, after, and during treatment. This list included questions such as "Am I radioactive?" "Will the treatments affect the rest of my body?" "Is radiation therapy a last resort?" "Do I have to be alone during the treatments?" and "How safe is the machine?" (Leahy, 1979).

Most of the books in this area suggested that the solution to the psychosocial and emotional problems of the patients is to have an attentive, sensitive, and supportive staff. A positive and appealing environment in both the waiting and treatment rooms is also suggested to help decrease the anxiety associated with the treatment. Regardless of all these suggestions pertaining to the outer environmental factors that affect the patient, I still have questions about the inner environment of the patient as he lies under the machine and how that could be affected and controlled.

Interviews with the treatment center's social worker and patients revealed that most patients view the treatments in a negative and apprehensive way. The most pervasive fear was that the machine with its tremendous power might harm healthy body tissue. One patient called the machine "the monster." Another patient said that she dreaded going to treatments, for the time spent under the machine, which might have been only a few minutes, was like an eternity as multiple fears raced through her mind. Most patients wished that the technician would count off the seconds aloud to help them through the sessions. The social worker related that the most difficult moment for many patients was the moment a loved one or friend who had accompanied them to the session had to leave. Most asked that someone remain in the room to the last possible moment. This fear of being alone in the room was common among the patients.

These fears, thoughts, emotions, feelings, and fantasies comprise the inner environment for many patients during treatment. This is an inner environment with which caregivers must be concerned. The patients need help to control the inner environment. The positive energies of this inner environment need to be harnessed not only to help the patient get through the treatment with greater ease and less anxiety but also to help the patient to fight against his disease as a partner with the radiotherapy. If the inner environment's negative energies need to be changed to positive energies, the question is, How can this best be done?

I believe that this process of affecting one's inner environment must begin before entering the treatment room, perhaps through one or more of the following methods:

   a. Prayer
   b. Visualization techniques
   c. Meditation
   d. Hynotherapy

For patients who wish to try these modes of achieving inner peace, a chaplain, social worker, and/or specialist in one of these therapies should be available at the radiotherapy unit. They could hold regularly scheduled group sessions, but they should also be available for private consultation before a specific patient enters treatment.

Prayer, for example, might work in the following way: In a group session, the chaplain would lead a discussion on prayer and its meaning for each of the patients. This discussion on the meaning of individual and personal prayer should direct the patient to understand and feel that prayer can function in two ways important for the state of his inner environment during therapy. Prayer can (a) help to change negative feelings into positive feelings by placing one into the care of a higher power and (b) give the patient a positive task to accomplish while under treatment, as prayers for health, healing, and recovery can be focused upon at that time. During group sessions, prayers from various faiths can be taught to those patients requesting such prayers. The emphasis, however, should be on the individual's power to pray from the heart, from the needs and feelings of the moment.

The chaplain can help group members to express their prayers and to practice the most effective way of saying them. The chaplain may want to combine therapeutic techniques such as visualization (the Simonton Method) or the use of fantasy as helpful techniques with the prayer experience. These groups should be held on a regular basis so that these patients can share their prayer experiences during treatment and can give added strength to each other.

The chaplain should make himself available to patients on an individual basis before they enter the treatment room. This individual attention might help reinforce what has been discussed in the group sessions. It might also be a way of helping a patient who is reaching out for help for the first time.

This method of group process and individual attention can be practiced for any of the therapeutic methods mentioned previously, as well as for others. Although ideally each therapeutic modality should have its own group of patients interested in using that method, the group sessions need not be so exclusive. A group session can teach the use of all these techniques. Although they differ from each other, they share very basic principles. The intention is to enable the patient to control his inner environment during treatment to achieve two goals: (1) to lessen the negative energies attached to the feelings of fear, anxiety, doubt, and loneliness that often are a part of the radiotherapy process and (2) to give the patient positive energies that will make him feel that he is helping to fight the disease. It is my belief that these therapeutic techniques in the radiotherapy unit will be of benefit not only to the patient but also to the staff in terms of having patients who approach their treatments with fewer fears and anxieties.

REFERENCES

Leahy, I.M. 1979. *The Nurse and Radiotherapy*. St. Louis: C.V. Mosby, p. 142.
Watson, J.C. 1974. *Patient Care and Special Procedures in Radiologic Technology*. St. Louis: C.V. Mosby, p. 191.

Chapter 5

RADIATION ONCOLOGY
Crossroad of Science and Soul
ISAMETTIN M. ARAL

I ncreased survival or cure rates have been obtained in patients with such malignancies as choriocarcinoma, childhood acute leukemia, and, perhaps, osteogenic sarcoma and non-Hodgkin's lymphoma. Unfortunately, there has been little improvement in survival or cure rates for patients with the more common malignancies of the lung, colon, prostate, and breast. The cure rate for the latter cancers has failed to change greatly within the past quarter-century.

The radiation therapy staff represents a conglomerate of professionals who have accepted by choice and/or necessity to aid the cancer patients in their physical and emotional needs and to comfort the families by attempting to lessen their worry, as well as by attempting to facilitate their coping with newly discovered social and economic stresses.

Radiation oncologists cannot be studied as a generalized group; rather, they must be divided into several subgroups, all of whom practice the same specialty but for varying reasons. For example, the general radiologist has elected to practice radiation therapy as a result of an insufficient number of radiotherapists in a given region or simply for financial gain. Certain radiotherapists' primary interest lies in radiobiological or radiophysical research, but they have made a decision to practice radiation therapy for practical reasons as well as financial ones. Finally, other individuals discover that the radiation therapy residency program is often less competitive than that for internal medicine or certain surgical subspecialties. Rather than remain general practitioners, the members of this group have chosen radiation therapy as their specialty. Although no data support this view, the author's belief, based on thirty years of practice, is that only 35 to 40 percent of radiotherapists have chosen this field because of an interest in the specific aspects of radiation therapy.

The radiation therapists, as well as their staffs, practice in a specialty of medicine where frustration is not uncommon, for a large percentage of their patients die within a relatively short period of time. Bronchogenic carcinoma, for example, is a malignancy whose victims will die within a period of nine to twelve months from the time of diagnosis. Yet, consolation can be derived from the fact that the physical suffering of the cancer patient can be eased through the use of radiation therapy. The bone pain frequently seen in patients with advanced carcinoma of the breast or prostate is often alleviated with small amounts of radiation. Bleeding in certain advanced gynecological or urinary malignancies also can often be controlled when other surgical or medical modalities become ineffective or impractical.

What makes the radiation oncology family choose to serve in what would seem to be a depressing field? Perhaps the ego is served because the respect of the community is bestowed upon those who are seen as "good guys" who altruistically help their fellow man. However, those working in the field of radiation oncology are not an exclusive fraternity endowed solely with divine inspiration; no doubt some intangible gratification does exist to make the profession desirable, as well as opportunities to excel because of limited competition and assured financial security (which is always gratifying). Radiation therapy also presents the practitioner with an opportunity to combat quackery. High vitamin and mineral therapy, as well as the intake of apricot and peach pit extracts, is the most obvious of these, but musculoskeletal manipulation, heliotherapy and hydrotherapy are also offered as cures for cancer. Radiation therapy has achieved a sophistication that has led to its competing on a common level with surgery and chemotherapy.

The radiation oncologist must maintain a balance between his work life and his family and social life. It is often said that the physician's family life deteriorates because of involvement with work and attachment to patients. In trying to help patients and their families, radiotherapists often do neglect their own families. No doubt the patient needs understanding and compassion, no doubt the patient's family looks for explanation, hope, and lessening of financial burden, but the radiation therapist must make time to live his own life, to care for his spouse, children, relatives, and friends. While patient care as well as professional competition consumes so much of the therapist's time that only a small percentage of therapists have both a successful professional and family life, a proper balancing of these obligations can make a radiotherapist a successful person.

Like the radiation therapist, the radiation therapy nurse and technician have often chosen the specialty because of its availability, limited competitiveness, financial security, and the opportunity to participate in easing the pain of the dying patient. Perhaps more than the radiotherapist, they are dealing day after day with the varied needs of the patient. It takes a special type of person to be able to comfort the sick. The constant struggle becomes traumatic and often expresses itself in severe psychological and psychosomatic ailments. In some areas, radiation oncology personnel are given vacations of up to ten weeks a year to allow time for physical and psychological recovery from exposure to radiation and cancer patients' psychological problems.

In summary, radiation oncologists working in a noble and difficult specialty deserve the understanding, recognition, and moral support that are necessary for their persevering in an effort to contribute to the physical and psychological welfare of those who are critically ill.

Chapter 6

THE WIDENING GAP BETWEEN THE SCIENCE AND THE ART OF PATIENT CARE IN RADIATION ONCOLOGY

HARRY L. BERMAN

Radiation oncology is involved with patients with malignant diseases, a group notable for its high degree of morbidity and mortality and therefore for its ability to disturb the quality of the patient's life. This discipline has evolved with great rapidity in the past fifteen years, its character changing from the empiricism of the past to greater scientific sophistication and accuracy. The resultant progress has enabled radiation therapists to measure and define parameters of treatment previously not susceptible to exact determination.

When unknown elements in the diagnosis and treatment of a disease are clarified by the availability of accurate means of measurement, the need for a theoretical or philosophical explanation to patients to cover gaps in knowledge vanishes or diminishes. As a consequence there may be a tendency on the part of physicians to ignore those abstract qualities not expressed in units of measurement and to leave patients and their families uninformed, or at least inadequately informed, about problems that loom as their greatest concerns. A simple schedule of daily appointments for a short period for treatment each day would seem to present no obstacles. In practice, it may not be that simple, and scheduling may pose annoying and upsetting difficulties.

Some basic features of radiation oncology play a role in the manner in which the psychosocial problems are confronted:

1. Radiation therapy, although it might be the sole method of definitive treatment for a given patient, is usually part of a program in which other members of a health care team participate. This raises questions about interdisciplinary relationships, definition of physician responsibilities, the role of paramedical individuals with interest in the psychosocial area, and the need for attention to many other functions.

2. It becomes apparent almost immediately in a course of radiation therapy that the treatment is something more than just matching a block of diseased tissue to a beam of radiation. The other needs of the patient are quickly made known to the radiologists, the nurses, the technologists, and even to the secretaries, the physicists, and the social workers. One may learn very early that the patient has transportation problems, concerns about nutrition, disruptions of family life, questions about medical costs, and a multiplicity of other worries. All of these may in some way affect the treatment program. Some may already have been taken care of by the primary care physician, by a hospital program attentive to the patient's psychosocial needs, by patients' supportive emotional attachments to their families, and by the fact that the overall requirements may be minimal. However, in no case can the radiologist be entirely exempt from dealing with these problems as they relate to the specialty of radiation oncology.

3. Radiation oncology is usually a hospital-based service that facilitates the availability of the needed psychosocial assistance. However, some practices are conducted in private offices, in which case the problems raised may be of such great proportion that they may interfere with the conduct of the professional care.

The services of radiation oncology may vary widely both quantatively and qualitatively in various places, not only from state to state and city to city but also from one section of a given city to another. These variations may be related to equipment, personnel, size of city, size and location of a hospital or private radiological office, quality of a medical staff, availability of total oncological professional services, quality of nursing and social service personnel, emphasis or lack thereof on teaching and research, presence or absence of university affiliation, and, finally, nature of the patient load. It is very difficult to establish standards of practice for proper radiation therapy for the entire country and to prescribe specifications for a given community. Oncologists are still in the process of examining patterns of care of cancer and trying to determine the best methods of treatment for particular cancers, not just radiological, but also surgical and medical and various combinations of these.

A broad spectrum of radiation therapy services exists today. At one end, where excellence is obvious, there is a financially well-supported university or university-affiliated medical center with capable representatives in all medical specialties. From them will come the many and varied patient referrals that will enable the radiation oncology service to have the necessary clinical material for maintaining the broad experience essential for its reputation for excellence. Available, too, will be the consultative skills and the supportive programs required for a well-coordinated team effort on behalf of the patient.

The radiation oncology department will have ample and varied modalities delivering radiation beams of different types, the adjunct instruments for treatment planning and dosimetry, a suitable budget, and the skilled personnel for performing the required tasks. It will have a residency training program and perhaps a school for the training of technologists. This department will likely have a busy research program, including participation in nationally organized protocols.

Needless to say, the administrative burdens of the chief of this department will be heavy. All the professional personnel will participate in extracurricular activities, not only in the hospital but also with the business and professional activities of local and national radiological organizations. Much of their time will be spent preparing the publications reporting the results of their research. One can conclude that little or no time will be available to them for looking after the psychosocial needs of their patients. This will have to be done by other persons.

At the other end of the spectrum is the medium-sized community hospital of 300 to 400 beds, possibly in a small city, where a board-certified therapeutic radiologist works with a single radiation therapy machine—perhaps cobalt 60—and treats twenty-five to thirty patients per day without the supportive services of a major center. His time will be limited, too, and will not be sufficient for looking after the psychosocial needs of every patient. His technologists may be helpful to him and he may get some help from the primary care physicians, but some of the responsibility cannot be avoided, and unless he deliberately makes a strong effort to limit his attentions in this area, he may find himself overwhelmed by his patients.

Other situations exist in which radiation therapy is administered. Limitations of medical care, especially in remote areas, may dictate the use of methods of treatment not considered ideal under optimum circumstances but representing the best available under the circumstances. This may be the case in a small town in an area at some distance from a properly staffed and equipped medical center. It is difficult to comment on what is right in this instance. The author has seen excellence prevail even though radiological therapy is rendered by a general radiologist who does therapy in addition to roentgen diagnosis. It might be argued that these patients would receive better care if they were transported to the larger center. However, proposed solutions may not be simple or acceptable because of pertinent obstacles, monumental human inertia, less than optimal concerns for patients' needs, nonavailability of suitable transportation or facilities for overnight housing, or the overwhelming pressure of medical costs. It should be apparent by now that good therapeutic radiology is egregiously expensive.

Radiation therapy is also administered as part of a private office practice. In doing accreditation surveys for the American College of Radiology, the author has seen some practices he considered to be excellent. One in particular, located near a major medical center, was a good example. The author raised a question about sending their patients to this easily accessible and obviously better equipped and staffed medical center and was advised that the patients preferred to be treated locally.

So far, radiation oncology has been considered as a *place* where a patient is treated. The author has always felt and shall continue to insist that radiation therapy is done not by a machine but more importantly by a physician, notably a radiologist. The two terms may not be synonymous. A dictum of the author's early days in radiation therapy stated that 60 percent of cancer patients had their fate determined by the natural history of their respective diseases, that 30 percent of cancer patients will be significantly affected by what their radiologists do or fail to do, and that for 10 percent of cancer patients the outcome will be determined by the machinery in use. This formula is now subject to revisions because of the progress made in radiation oncology, but the functions and importance of the radiation therapist have not diminished.

Since the role of the radiation oncologist is not inconsequential, what kind of person should take on this role? Aside from professional competence, are there desirable personal requisites for one to practice this specialty? In trying to answer this question, one who is a radiologist must be certain that he is not looking into a mirror. Generally, radiation oncologists will be a cross section of the medical profession, and no one type can be seen as the proper model. They will be judged by peers in radiology, by medical and surgical colleagues, by patients, and by associates in administrative affiliations. Their perceptions of the radiation oncologist will affect the solidity of his appointment to any position, the referral of patients, and the relationships with patients. All of these relationships may be consistently smooth for some individuals and perversely tempestuous for others. Ideally, the achievements of a radiation oncology department in meeting prescribed professional objectives, while satisfying the needs and requirements of its patients, will be the measure of success. It is well known that the personal qualities of the radiation oncologist are important elements in the level of success attained.

Although one measure of proficiency for a radiation oncologist is Radiology Board certification, it is not the sole yardstick. Board certification may not be matched by excellence in the application of knowledge to the actual performance of methods of treatment. The author participated in the peer review of a fellow radiotherapist in his home area conducted by the state medical society. He came to the attention of this committee because of his involvement in several medical malpractice suits. In the course of the investigation the committee found multiple examples of bad judgment and deficiencies in his conduct of radiation therapy. Nevertheless, most of the patients who were interviewed thought highly of him and praised him as a fine physician. It was obvious that his convincing, articulate manner of speech with a well-modulated voice had been used to impress his patients and to compensate for the shortcomings in his medical knowledge. What may be a useful attribute for a used-car salesman is not necessarily desirable for the care of cancer patients. Comforting reassurance to a patient and family may have its merits but not at the price of inexcusably poor medical care.

This is not to suggest that one has only a single choice between two options. A considerate, compassionate, sincere attitude on the part of the radiation oncologist—always associated with demonstrable interest in the patient, with measured objectivity, and without undue subjectivity—is ideally a proper position for him to assume. However, as indicated earlier, the increasing preoccupation of the radiation oncologist with the scientific parameters in the management of patients with malignant disease will interfere with devoting efforts towards an optimum concern for the psychosocial aspects. The need for establishing priorities for the available time will require the delegation of responsibilities in the latter area to qualified individuals other than radiologists.

Chapter 7

THE X-RAY THERAPY WAITING ROOM
More Than That

SUCHA O. ASBELL

T he waiting rooms of departments of radiation therapy
provide the following:

1. A place for patients and their families to be seated
2. A time for anticipation before treatment or visit with the physician
3. Opporuntity for patient and family to converse with the nurse
4. Opportunity for patient and family to converse with other patients
5. Opportunity for patient and family to converse with other patients' families

Perhaps more important than these, however, is the education or miseducation of patients and their families regarding cancer and its treatment.

In the late 1960s, patients were just beginning to be informed of their diagnoses. At that time, the general public was less informed than now about cancer, and most people believed that all cancers were incurable. If a person had a malignant disease, he feared being ostracized by friends and family if they learned of his illness. The word *cancer* was taboo, never to be used; the disease was not to be discussed, as if the more said about it, the more likely the patient's demise. Many believed cancer to be contagious and also feared that patients receiving CO^{60} or radiation therapy were radioactive.

41

It is understandable why the waiting room in many institutions discouraged patients' discussing their diagnosis and treatment. Physicians feared that patients learning their diagnosis or seeing other patients suffering with nausea or alopecia would quit before receiving full treatment.

As a consequence, the inception of a group dynamics movement for the waiting room constituency was delayed until the early 1970s when patients were first advised of their diagnoses. As this was permitted, the public became better informed and better educated. That part of the uninformed public in the waiting room of a radiation therapy department, however, was quickly converted to becoming knowledgeable about cancer, the role of radiation therapy, and its palliative or curative ability and sequelae. Patients reconfirmed information from their doctors with other patients and/or their families. Although occasionally incorrect information was transmitted or facts distorted, more frequently, patients and their families received reconfirmation of the facts relayed to them by their doctors. Thus, satisfaction and contentment with the management that had been scheduled was re-established. Occasionally, new patients would formally request consultation with patients who had already gone through the ordeal of radiation therapy. Doctors, noting fear in their patients, would suggest discussion with previous patients in the hope of alleviating anxiety.

Efforts of doctors, paramedics, and the American Cancer Society helped remove some of the erroneous beliefs about cancer, but the discussions in the waiting room provided patients and their families with answers to questions regarding the fine details of what to anticipate from the disease, its treatment, and its side effects.

Physicians trained before the 1960s might still tell their patients, "Don't listen to anything you hear in the waiting room, just listen to me." Comparing the treatments for different tumors and their side effects can lead to a patient's insecurity. Seeing patients weekly provides the physician with some assurance of being able to correct any misinformation or misinterpretation of treatment policy or sequelae. For example, patients coming in for management of cancer of the breast, one being postmastectomy and the other having inflammatory cancer, would not understand the differences in treatment of their malignancies. They would need explanations of established treatments and of differences in management of their diseases.

There was once a sign in the author's department stating, "Don't Discuss Your Diagnosis With Other Patients." This sign was virtually ignored by all. Patients cannot be expected not to interact with one another when placed together for fifteen minutes to one hour. The division of the waiting room—follow-up patients from regular daily patients under treatment—led to a noticeable increase in the number of malcontent patients receiving daily treatments. The presence of patients who have had previous experience with radiation therapy provides stability to the waiting room group's interaction and adds a feeling of hope in regard to the potential for successful treatment of cancer by radiation therapy. Diminished anxiety, opportunity of treatment, and appreciation of the physician are learned from those experienced patients who have returned to the radiation therapy waiting room. Their presence is helpful when the physician is delayed in the operating room or is with a very sick patient. The value of seeing the doctor gains importance and is noted as "being worth waiting for."

Also present are patients or family members who will assist other patients to and from the bathroom or bring them coffee. Providing other patients with coffee and tea gives patients something to do while waiting and provides a renewal of energy when there has been an unexpected delay. Often a very sick patient waiting his turn will have a treatment earlier and out of turn because of the thoughtfulness of a more fortunate patient or one who has already been through similar circumstances.

The author has been separating the very ill inpatients from those who are relatively well into two waiting areas. When well patients see someone very ill or hear cries of pain, they may become disturbed. Emotionally and mentally disturbed patients and patients with difficult personalities usually attract a nurse's attention. It is her responsibility to learn the problems and comprehend the situation. Separating these patients from the more stable ones provides a better atmosphere for everyone.

A "sign-in" procedure allows physicians to know how long patients have been waiting and assists them in taking the patients in proper order. Before this method was adopted, arguments occurred between patients over who had come first and who should be seen first.

Good waiting room tactics should be shared. Learning from the conduct of other physicians across the country could help to provide a better milieu for patients and reinforce the support being given to this special patient population, both therapeutically and psychosocially.

Chapter 8

STRATEGIES FOR ASSISTING PATIENTS TO COPE WITH CANCER

Y. MARUYAMA AND S. A. TAUSEND

C ancer diagnoses are known to threaten the patient's medical, social, psychological, and economic well-being (Cullen, 1976; Healy, 1970; Hinton, 1970; Quint, 1965; Rosillo et al., 1973), and these threats often are shared by persons close to the patient, e.g. family, friends, relatives, co-workers, and acquaintances (Goffman, 1963; Holland, 1973; Kitsuse, 1980). Thus, over the past decade increasing attention has been given within medical contexts to assisting patients to cope with the psychosocial as well as the medical aspects of cancer (Blumberg et al., 1980; Cullen, 1976; Holland, 1973; Vettessee, 1976; Weisman, 1979).

This chapter focuses on the fact that the physician and staff can "set the tone for successful coping or not during the cancer patient's therapy" (Blumberg et al., 1980). Specifically, the chapter describes strategies in use at the University of Kentucky Radiation Therapy Oncology Center to assist the patient's psychosocial adjustment to cancer. With most cancer patients, the greater the likelihood of complete cure, the more rapid the rehabilitation process, including initial psychosocial adjustment to the disease. The lesser the likelihood of cure and the greater the malignancy of the cancer, the greater the task of the physician and the medical staff to help the patient adapt to the disease (Sutherland and Orbach, n.d.; Weisman and Worden, 1977). Hence, at present the strategies are directed primarily at the

45

"average" cancer patient undergoing treatment at the center.

Unique factors of the state and patient population that affect the authors' clinic and procedures will be described. In particular, the effect on clinic procedures of professionals dealing with a population that tends to be diverse but sometimes low in income and education and drawn primarily from rural areas with regional language and subcultural differences will be noted. Second, the role structure of the clinic staff and the physical arrangement of the clinic in relation to psychosocial adjustment goals will be described. Specific attention is drawn to considering the importance of communication of medical information as a triangulation procedure between physician, patient, and staff members. In addition, the value of arranging the therapeutic setting to encourage a patient-to-patient support system is discussed.

THE SETTING

The University of Kentucky Radiation Oncology Center

The central and eastern regions of Kentucky are characterized by numerous small, cohesive communities serving a widely dispersed population. The region contains an inadequate number of physicians or health care specialists necessary for tertiary care. Instead, the residents of central and eastern Kentucky are referred to medical facilities in the major urban communities of the state (Ford, 1964; Friedl, 1978) for their tertiary health care services.

Over the past decade the University of Kentucky Radiation Therapy Oncology Center has been recognized as a major cancer treatment center in the state (Maruyama, 1977). It is both recognized and supported by the National Cancer Institute as a regional treatment facility and research center. Announcement of the NCI support in 1975 was accompanied by extensive publicity in the mass media, which created a positive view of the center for Kentucky residents.* In addition, as a University Hospital for the

---

*UK Uses Atomic Radiation for Cancer Treatment, Louisville *Courier Journal,* February 3, 1975; Medical Center Designated Special Cancer Facilty, Lexington *Herald Leader,* August 21, 1975.

Commonwealth of Kentucky, the center is viewed as offering the best of current medical practices and multidisciplinary care as well as being on the forefront of cancer research and development in the state.† Thus, patients referred to the center anticipate the best of current care procedures and usually express confidence in the medical treatment procedures suggested by the attending physicians.

The positive image of the center within the state also appears to be reinforced via the strong kin-based system of human relations prevalent in Kentucky. The central and eastern regions of the state are characterized by small cohesive communities with close, caring families. The ill health of any member becomes of general concern to all family and community members, most of whom offer support to the patient. From the center's perspective, one unusual manifestation of such a kin-based system is the desire of multiple family members to participate in decisions for care of the cancer patients and to be involved in the treatment process. As a result, patients who are treated at the center (and their accompanying family members) become a potent force when they return to the community and qualitatively evaluate the medical and nonmedical care received. A measure of the center's effectiveness thus is found through the continued confidence of new patients in services offered at the center.

Patient Population

The distribution of medical conditions seen at the University of Kentucky Radiation Therapy Oncology Center appears to differ from patient populations at many other similar treatment centers. The patient population includes an unusually large proportion of female gynecological malignancies, lung cancers, and central nervous system tumors. The center's case load contains the usual proportions of breast, bowel, head and neck, childhood, and metastatic cancers, leukemias, lymphomas, and genitourinary tract malignancies. With a large fraction of female cancer

---

†New Forms of Cancer Treatment Being Tried at UK, Lexington *Herald Leader*, June 12, 1977.

patients, sexual differences in adaptation to disease are also important (Leigh et al., 1980). Presumably, each of these cancers will entail individual differences in patient adaptation. However, currently certain basic psychosocial considerations common to all cancer cases (Holland, 1973; Weisman, 1979) are assumed to operate.

Clearly, the overwhelming concern of all cancer patients is the hope that the condition is surgically removable and curable. Virtually as important, but often less obvious, are the fears of the patients based on generalized and often erroneous beliefs about cancer as a disease, which may or may not apply to their cases. Included are fears of mutilation or disfigurement, of severe symptomatology, of painful progression of disease, of bleeding, of difficulty breathing or swallowing, of nausea and vomiting, and of loss of limb, body parts, scalp hair, or mental competence and the overriding fear that death is imminent (Blumberg et al., 1980; Holland, 1973; Vettessee, 1976). One fear openly expressed among our patients is that cancer is contagious. Yet, despite these fears, which may be exacerbated by the limited education of many central and eastern Kentucky residents, most of the center's patients are committed to wage the maximal effort within their emotional and financial capabilities to cooperate with the physician and medical staff to achieve the therapeutic goal of cure or tumor control. Some factors in patient coping strategies are shown in Table 8-I.

Table 8-I
FACTORS IN PATIENT STRATEGIES IN COPING

- Type of Cancer
- Age
- Sex
- Marital Status/Child
- Socioeconomic
- Emotional Reaction
- Family/Friends
- Community
- Medical/Therapy
- Religious
- Alcohol/Drugs
- Adaptation

STRATEGIES TO MAXIMIZE PSYCHOSOCIAL ADJUSTMENT TO CANCER: ROLE STRUCTURE OF STAFF

The authors believe that to reduce the initial psychosocial stress of cancer, the goals of the primary care radiotherapist and staff should be as follows: Each patient should be assisted to (a) perceive realistically his own diagnosis, (b) maintain a positive self-image, and (c) preserve somatic and psychological integrity. To accomplish these goals, the authors have concentrated on developing the role structure between staff members to increase patient communication and have arranged the clinic physically to decrease psychosocial stress. Some coping strategies are shown in Table 8-II.

Staff Role Structure

General Staff Procedures

The entire staff of the center is trained to recognize that each interaction with the patients and their families may be a positive or negative encounter affecting future care decisions not only for those individuals but for the broader community they represent. Consequently, the center's staff strives to create a general atmosphere that is pleasant, positive, supportive, and concerned with the patient's medical and nonmedical needs. Within this framework, roles can be tightly structured but highly interrelated, as described later, especially concerning the communication of medical information.

Table 8-II
COPING STRATEGY

- Emotional Reaction
- Friends/Family
- Doctor
- Therapy
- Cancer Clinic Personnel
- Defining Plight
- Intervention

The Radiotherapist

Physicians at the center must be cognizant of several features of the doctor-patient relationship that potentially act as barriers to interacting with residents from central and eastern Kentucky. First, the health belief system of many of these Kentucky residents includes an attitude of stoicism toward illness and injury, which frequently includes aspects of religious fatalism (Friedl, 1978). As a consequence, the patient and his family may listen stoically to a medical explanation of the disease and to the treatment recommendations without fully processing the content of the communication. Despite the physician's effort to discuss each case and treatment recommendation as positively as possible using language that appears to be understood by the patient and interpreting medical terms, the communication gap imposed by cultural differences toward illness may hinder such efforts, however well meaning.

A second unusual factor for the physician in dealing with some of the center's cancer patients is the social barrier erected by folk beliefs about proper behavior in medical settings. In kin-based systems, the authority structure of the family frequently extends to extrafamilial settings, such as with the physician. In such cases, the patient may consider it improper to ask for clarification of an unclear statement or term and also may mask his actual response to the presentation of information about the disease or treatment. Furthermore, due to authority beliefs, the patient is as likely to be influenced by the physician's sincerity and demeanor as by the content of the communication. Hence, it is essential that the physician convey acceptance of the patient and the disease and respect for any obvious cultural differences. Center staff encourages patients to ask questions of the physician and also of the nurse and other staff members.

A third factor the physician must consider at the center is the intense self-reliance of residents, especially those from some of the more remote Kentucky regions. Patients appearing at the center frequently feel chagrined that their self-doctoring has failed (Hocstrasser and Nickerson, 1966) and that they must seek specialized medical care. The physician especially may elicit a potentially negative response from patients when the likelihood of help is small or when care recommendations require large expenses, especially if assistance will be needed through social services (Stekert, 1970).

Given the preceding factors, the radiotherapist's key role is that of conveying to the patient confidence in the recommended treatment program and in the quality and importance of care available at the center. While the physician monitors all aspects of the patient's treatment program, important communication support comes from the staff members of the center. Direct and open communication with each patient to interpret various aspects of the information presented is often best accomplished by the staff. The close cooperation between physician and staff aids the patients in initial decision making associated with treatment and their progress through therapy.

The Clinic Nurse

At the center, the patient's initial in-depth interaction is with a clinic nurse selected for regionally appropriate communication skills. During this encounter, the nurse obtains a brief history and examines the patient's vital signs. The center favors matching nurses and patients from Kentucky, as they share similar language patterns, behaviors, and regional jargon. By immediately establishing a line of similarity between the patient and a member of the professional staff at the center, the unfamiliarity and attendant fear of a medical treatment center and the barriers that potentially can arise from medical personnel can be reduced (Fabrega, 1970; Kleinman, 1980).

Following the initial interview, the patients generally trust the staff to interpret the recommendations of the doctor and to assist in reviewing the decision-making aspects of the treatment if they feel it is necessary.

Simulation and Simulator Technologist

Once treatment is accepted, patients in the clinic are eager to commence therapy but may be surprised by the pretreatment procedures required. In explaining the need for precision and accuracy in radiotherapy, center staff strives to impress the patient with the power of modern medical technology and the skill of the staff that controls the treatment procedures. Hence, the anxiety the patient may feel is transformed to confidence in learning the steps of the treatment program.

In the simulation step, consents are signed, contours obtained, and ports are set on the patient. An attentive and sympathetic technologist who is sensitive to the patient's anxiety begins the therapeutic process by explaining positioning and carefully and accurately placing the skin marks under radiographic control, and in so doing explains the steps and timing of the therapeutic process. CT scanning and mold or immobilizer construction also may be scheduled at this time and their significance explained.

Radiation Therapy Technology Staff

The staff in radiation therapy plays a critical and essential role in decreasing the patient's psychosocial stress. The frequent, daily treatment visits allow a close and friendly relationship to develop easily and naturally between technologist and patient. The patients (all of whom seem readily to understand the authority structure of the clinic) are more relaxed with the technologist and turn to him for advice on both medical and nonmedical matters. The technologist may be the first to know of the patient's need for medication, to explain the common symptoms associated with treatment, and to evaluate tissue reactions. By promptly responding to these problems or referring the problems promptly, the technologist is perceived by the patient as a person who is concerned and competent.

The therapist and the staff begin to establish a relationship with the patient by introducing him to the machines that represent the center's standard therapy equipment. In this clinic a machine may be given a personal name as a means of reducing its intimidating nature, but more important, by familiarly discussing the machine and explaining its operation and the normal reactions to radiation, the technologist encourages the patient to relate to the machine as a positive component of the therapy program. This procedure appears to reduce the patient's concern about the operation of the machines, and the treatment sessions rapidly become routine. The therapist discusses the treatment prescription and program; the technologist makes the prescription a reality.

A measure of the success of the center's technologists occurs through the mementos and gifts in appreciation of services and care that may be left by patients at the end of the treatment process. Ending treatment conducted by a particularly sensitive and caring technologist may be a moment of sadness for the patient.

Clinical Physics/Treatment Planning Staff

The demands placed on accurate and precise radiation therapy have created an environment of great responsibility with attendant stresses upon the center's technologist staff. In addition, the great variety of treatments used, e.g. arcs, bolus, compensators, hemi-body, total body, wedge pairs, electron beam, irregular fields, total nodal, mantle, inverted Y, hockey stick, mini-mantle, rotational, and super-fractionated schedule, rems, rets, and so forth, requires constant attention to detail by the radiotherapy treatment staff. Any deviations, however minor, from schedules, dose/day, dose/fraction, dropped appointments, and the like, become a source of tremendous anxiety to the staff. The center has developed a clinical physics/treatment planning staff (Maruyama and Herring, 1979) who, due to a great deal of technical, physical, dosimetric knowledge and their proficiency, greatly support the technological staff. In addition, simulation and frequent port films verification allow the technologist (or one who fills in when another is away) a real means of reassurance, sustaining their and the patients' confidence in accuracy. Regular chart surveillance and audits further ensure that the treatment prescription is rendered accurately, exactly as prescribed.

MACHINES

The authors have observed that the large, imposing modern machines that represent the standard equipment in the department have a positive but intimidating effect on the cancer patient. The initial encounter with and introduction to the machine represent an experience wherein the patient's concern about his disease is transferred to the power of modern technology and to the radiation therapists, physicists, and technologists who seem to control those powerful rays. At the same time, it is a frightening experience. To reduce this anxiety, some of the center's machines have names (such as Henry), which allow patients to relate in a more familiar and friendly way with them. The patients do seem to lose their anxieties about the machines, and the brief treatment sessions soon become simply another routine. The treatment prescription (number of treatments) soon begins to represent a beginning and a reasonable end point in which to fit the therapeutic effort.

SOCIAL SERVICES

The great concern and anxieties about details and means for obtaining care are greatly aided by the availability of an effective support social services program. Housing, means of travel, assistance, and economics are some of the areas discussed, which greatly allays patient anxiety. Questions concerning housing, means of travel, economic assistance, and social support are raised and evaluated by these adjunct staff members. An inventory of some common concerns is shown in Table 8-III, and to address these problems, a social service worker is promptly available.

PHYSICAL ARRANGEMENTS AT THE CLINIC TO REDUCE PSYCHOSOCIAL STRESS

Waiting Rooms

At this center, multiple widely spaced waiting rooms were

Table 8-III
INVENTORY OF CONCERNS

- Health
- Work
- Finances
- Family
- Friends
- Disability
- Existential
- Self

designed to segregate specific categories of patients from each other. Those with certain categories of diagnoses (e.g. gynecologic) are clustered in specific areas near the related treatment machines. Others with, for example, head and neck, lung, and palliative problems tend to cluster in other areas. This general plan and design of the department places similar patients together and reduces the stress engendered by encountering patients who exceed the patient's own level of illness, disfigurement, or psychological malfunctioning.

Encouraging Patient-to-Patient Support

Within each waiting area of the clinic, the furniture is arranged to encourage small group interaction. (Individual chairs separated from the group are also provided for patients who wish to sit alone.) Patients may sit in these groups and chat while awaiting their treatment time. All patients, whether of high or low performance status, are very much in need of companionship, group identity, and peer support (Schmale, 1972), and the opportunity offered by waiting areas appears to offer a positive setting for the radiotherapy clinic.

Patient-to-patient interaction reinforces staff explanations of the treatment process and markedly assists in altering new patients' views to a more realistic perception of their diseases. In addition, the patients are very effective in socializing one another into the milieu of the clinic. For example, patients instruct one another on the reputations of the physicians ("nice," "very courteous," "too busy," "the favorite"), technologists ("talks a lot," "kind," "has good jokes"), and other staff members. Even patients who do not enter into the conversations, but only listen, still appear to respond positively to the information shared by the group.

Patients' feelings of hopelessness are gradually altered to acceptance of the diagnosis and the treatments that are necessary, and those who become more advanced in their treatment course begin to talk to those who have just started. During follow-up clinic visits, many patients return to visit their machines and technologists. If the course of disease is proceeding favorably and if there are other patients with similar conditions present, the patient may be encouraged to volunteer a word of support and explanation. Receiving this information from an experienced but similarly afflicted patient appears greatly to aid and comfort the patient who is involved in a similar course of therapy. Thus, patients provide considerable support to each other. Patient-to-patient contact reinforced by the technologists and radiotherapists represent a distinctly positive factor in this clinic.

DISCUSSION AND CONCLUSION

Adaptive mechanisms of patients in dealing with the diagnosis of cancer or chronic disease have been described. It has been of some interest to the authors that the immediate reaction of a patient given the diagnosis of cancer is one of prompt depression, strong denial, and the certain fear that death is directly forthcoming (Schmale, 1972). This reaction is very much shared by persons close to the patient, i.e. family, friends, relatives, associates, colleagues, and acquaintances. The psychological mechanism of coping with the diagnosis of cancer and adjusting to the disease is very closely related with the physician and his staff and the possibility of treatment offered to the patient. The possibility of medical therapy for these dreaded diseases allows the patient to cope with the diagnosis of cancer. The role of the radiation therapists and their staffs in this adaptive process has been observed in the University of Kentucky Radiation Therapy Oncology Center and can be a positive and effective one.

The authors believe, as has been well stated, for example, by Kennedy (1973), that "all health practitioners must learn the covert assumptions and basic reasoning patterns of their clients. Health professionals are interpreters and intermediaries between a body of scientific knowledge about health enhancement and the realities of folk medicine, primitive medicine, and public safety practice within any given community. To render a valuable and effective professional service the . . . professional . . . must master both worlds of thought and behavior. He must know how providers think and behave; and he must know how clients believe and act." These factors relate importantly to the radio-therapist but equally importantly to the clinical staff.

In current cancer therapy, radiotherapy represents an important component of cancer treatment in approximately 50 percent of cancer patients. At the University of Kentucky, approximately 1,000 patients per year are seen in radiation oncology and treated for a variety of malignant diseases. Since radiotherapy plays an extremely important role in the treatment of these conditions, radiation therapy plays an important role in the coping strategy offered by the medical center for the patient with cancer. Thus, the design and organization of the clinic and treatment facility and the attitudes and concerns of the clinic personnel are very important to the psychosocial adaptation of the patient to his disease.

The emotional reaction of the cancer patient appears to respond to the therapeutic environment and creates a setting wherein psychosocial intervention is potentially usable; however, many factors appear to be important for such a program. This makes for a difficult problem not easily addressable in this clinic at the present time. The problem is of sufficient complexity that without further in-depth and long-range study, an effective program will not be possible. The clinic generally tends to segregate patients by performance status, and this seems to aid patient adaptation. However, other factors such as friends and family, group, and community attitude appear to play an important role. In Kentucky, cancer patients have special psychosocial problems that appear to require further careful investigation, and the development of interventional programs would be desirable.

REFERENCES

Blumberg, B., M. Flaherty, and J. Lewis, eds. 1980. *Coping with Cancer.* Washington, D.C.: National Cancer Institute.

Cullen, J.W., ed. 1976. *Cancer: The Behavioral Dimensions.* New York: Raven Press.

Fabrega, H., Jr. 1970. Dynamics of Medical Practice in a Folk Community. *Milbank Memorial Fund Quarterly,* 48:391-412.

Ford, T.R. 1964. *Health and Demography in Kentucky.* Lexington, Kentucky: University of Kentucky Press.

Friedl, J. 1978. *Health Care Service and the Appalachian Migrant.* Washington, D.C.: Department of Health, Education, and Welfare.

Goffman, E. 1963. *Stigma: Notes on the Management of Spoiled Identity.* Englewood Cliffs, New Jersey: Prentice-Hall.

Healy, J.E., Jr., ed. 1970. *Ecology of the Cancer Patient: Proceedings of Three Interdisciplinary Conferences on Rehabilitation of the Patient with Cancer.* Washington, D.C.: The Interdisciplinary Communication Association.

Hinton, J. 1970. Bearing Cancer. *British Journal of Medical Psychology, 46:*105-113.

Hocstrasser, D. and G. Nickerson. 1966. Community Health Work in Southern Appalachia. *Mountain Life and Work, 42:*8-16.

Holland, J.F. 1973. Psychologic Aspects of Cancer. In J.F. Holland and E. Frei, III, eds., *Cancer Medicine.* Philadelphia: Lea and Febiger, pp. 991-1021.

Kennedy, D. 1973. Perceptions of Illness and Healing. *Social Science and Medicine, 7:*787-805.

Kitsuse, J.I. 1980. Coming Out All Over: Deviants and the Politics of Social Problems. *Social Problems, 28:*1-13.

Kleinman, A. 1980. *Patients and Healers in the Context of Culture.* Berkeley, California, University of California Press.

Leigh, H., J. Ungera, and B. Percarpio. 1980. Denial and Helplessness in Cancer Patients Undergoing Radiation Therapy: Sex Differences and Implications for Prognosis. *Cancer, 45:* 3086-89.

Maruyama, Y. 1977. A Special Radiation Oncology Center for Research into Cancer Treatment and Diagnosis. *Journal of Kentucky Medical Association,* 75:222,

Maruyama, Y. and D. Herring. 1979. Survey of Treatment- Planning Personnel in Radiotherapy. *Applied Radiology, 8:* 51-57.

Quint, J. 1965. Institutionalized Practices for Information Control. *Psychiatry,* 28:119-32.

Rosillo, R.H., M.J. Welty, and W.P. Graham. 1973. The Patient with Maxillofacial Cancer II— Psychological Aspects. *Nursing Clinics of North America, 8:* 153-158.

Schmale, A.H. 1972. Giving Up As a Final Common Pathway to Changes in Health. *Advances in Psychosomatic Medicine, 8:* 20-40.

Stekert, J. 1970. Focus for Conflict: Southern Mountain Medical Beliefs in Detroit. *Journal of American Folklore, 83:*115-56.

Sutherland, A.M. and C.E. Orbach. n.d. Depressive Reactions Associated with Surgery for Cancer. In *Psychological Impact of Cancer,* American Cancer Society, Professional Education Publications, pp. 17-21.

Vettessee, J.M. 1976. Problems of the Patient Confronting the Diagnosis of Cancer. In J.W. Cullen et al., eds., *Cancer: The Behavioral Dimension,* New York: Raven Press, pp. 275-82.

Weisman, A.D. 1979. *Coping with Cancer.* New York: McGraw- Hill.

Weisman, A.D. and J.W. Worden. 1977. The Existential Plight in Cancer: Significance of the First 100 Days. *International Journal of Psychiatry in Medicine, 7:*1-15.

Chapter 9

THE RADIATION ONCOLOGIST IN PRIVATE PRACTICE
A Personal Point of View

ARNOLD WALD

I am a radiation oncologist practicing full-time in a private office. I have been using high energy radiation therapy equipment (cobalt 60) to treat cancer patients since 1961, or for more than twenty years. My major goal has been to deliver optimum radiation therapy to the patients in my county. I do not consider myself a pioneer or innovator in the "death and dying" movement, in the "emotional care of cancer patients" movement, or in the "healing of the healers" movement.

As a radiation oncologist, my role has not been that of a researcher or developer of new ideas. I have not been involved extensively in clinical therapy trials. Rather, as an observer and synthesizer, I have attempted to pick out the best radiotherapeutic techniques and concepts for the management of each type of cancer and apply these principles and methods at my community level to day-to-day patient care. I have regularly attended local, regional, and national radiation oncology meetings and seminars to learn to choose the best techniques of or combinations of radiation therapy, chemotherapy, and surgery. In the early years of my radiotherapy practice, I was unaware (certainly on a conscious level) of many of the emotional reactions of my patients to their initial diagnosis of cancer, of its impact on their interpersonal relations, of the patient's fears of surgery, radiation therapy, and chemotherapy, and of the patient's feelings of loss of self or of body image. Nor was I often aware of the patients' fear of death when they were diagnosed as having cancer, even when the cancer was early and curable. "Denial" had not yet been discovered, so of course none of my patients needed to deny anything. Nor did I.

I was a typical narrowly oriented physician trained in a large New York City medical school to (1) save lives, (2) cure cancer (or whatever illness afflicted my patients), (3) be *objective* when it came to patients and not to let personal feelings get in the way of taking care of acutely ill patients or patients with disgusting tumors, with ugly, deformed bodies, or with offensive personalities. I was taught to be kind, understanding, compassionate, all-accepting, all-loving, nonjudgmental, and fair in treating all sick people equally, carefully, and considerately. I *never got angry*. Giving was the goal, the ideal. The harder I worked, the more I sacrificed, the more selfless I became, the better the doctor I was, and of course, being the good doctor was the highest ideal.

I bought it all, the whole damn package. I was the typical compulsive hardworking physician; my patients and practice came first; everything important, my wife, my family, my friends, and I, was second.

The result was a busy, successful practice, but a personal life that was less and less satisfying. I had difficulties in my marriage, I did not really know my children or get close to them, and I did not know or understand what was going wrong. After all, I was doing everything right, yet it did not work for me. The solution was not instantaneous or easy. It has taken years and still is not quite complete.

The keys to changing the pattern that I was stuck in were (1) realizing that something was wrong and (2) admitting it to myself and appreciating how bad things really were. Then through a painfully slow process of personal therapy, self-examination, and growth, I learned to become aware of and to recognize the inner person within me. Then I learned to accept and trust this inner person. Finally, I have been able to integrate my inner person's needs and abilities, to become a more human health caregiver. As my personal therapy and growth progressed, I became open to new ideas about aspects of medical care that had been unfamiliar, particularly with respect to the emotional and psychologic needs of patients and of caregiver. I enrolled in and participated in many workshops, meetings, and seminars dealing with the emotional and psychologic aspects of health care of patients with cancer. The effect of this new state of personal awareness has been to alter profoundly my methods of practice and my understanding of the patient's problems (much to the better) and also to enable me to evolve more comprehensive programs using supporting staff members to deal with the multitude of emotional, social, and psychologic problems that my cancer patients were experiencing. I was able to give up control of many aspects of patient care. It has enabled me to find a richness in patient contacts, to deal more effectively with the pain and stresses that a radiotherapeutic practice must involve one in, and to find an enriched personal life that balances the toil and strain involved in practice. Most important, by learning to accept the limitations of my radiotherapeutic modality, I could become closer to patients without necessarily becoming responsible for bad outcomes and/or their deaths.

I would like to describe how my practice has evolved through various phases during which I have tried different methods of psychologic and social support for my patients. Some of these methods have been only marginally successful, others have failed, but by the process of trial and error, a practice format has now evolved that is improving the comprehensive nature of patient care and at the same time reducing strain on the caregiver. None of my office programs was funded by outside sources or grants; all were supported by income from the private practice or were at times done on a volunteer basis. My first project involved hiring a doctoral candidate psychologist to meet with cancer patients whom I perceived to be in need. Prior to instituting this program, we conducted a survey to determine the emotional care needs of patients being treated in my office. In response to a questionnaire distributed to these patients, we found that more than 60 percent indicated some need for psychologic care and support. Once the program was started, however, and in trying to guide and direct patients to the psychologist, we had a very low patient acceptance rate, less than 5 percent. Of those who had an initial visit, less than half continued with one or more follow-up visits. The psychologist worked four hours a week during 1975 and half of 1976. The few patients who availed themselves of the psychologist's services received considerable benefit in their personal lives and in the management of their cancer. After one and a half years, this program was discontinued because it was helping only a small proportion of the total number of cancer patients that were being treated in the radiotherapy practice.

In 1976 and 1977, a nurse counselor was hired on a part-time basis. Her training following graduation from nursing school included a bachelor of science degree in psychology. She worked under the supervision of a psychiatrist who was a volunteer. The nurse's interest was directed principally to the psychologic aspects of patient care, and she saw many patients on a continuing basis and was able to provide significant psychologic support for them and their families. Her part-time work (two days a week) and her total time availability were insufficient. She met with patients just one day per week, and there was not ample office space for her to have a regular meeting room with patients. In addition, her interest in social service problems, nutritional support, transportation, and financial problems of patients was not keen, and she was only able to provide psychologic counseling rather than the more comprehensive care that the patients required.

During her employment, we made serious attempts to organize and operate group therapy for cancer patients with the participation of the volunteer psychiatrist, as well as the nurse. I, too, attended most of the patient group sessions. During the period that this program was in effect, there were many worthwhile group meetings for the patients, but the attempt failed because we were trying to fit the patients into a treatment plan and method that the patients were not able to accept. I believe that my presence was counterproductive to more open group meetings.

Another plan that was tried was the use of group meetings for the radiation therapy office staff. The entire spectrum of the staff was included—the radiation oncologist, radiation technologists, x-ray technicians, secretaries, typists, receptionists, business office personnnel, and so forth. The sessions were conducted at the end of a working day, every other week for approximately three months. These group meetings were partially successful in that the office staff, in general, was brought into a more active participation in understanding the patient's needs and problems and the strains that the professional staff in the office was undergoing. The staff members were able to develop a better feeling of camaraderie and support for each other, as well as for the patient. However, the staff group failed when we attempted to have the meetings go beyond the superficial feelings and considerations. Revealing personal feelings on a deeper level was too threatening, and after three months, as attendance fell off, the office groups were discontinued. The nurse herself became "burned out." Working with cancer and dying patients was too emotionally painful and charged for her, and she eventually left the position in the radiotherapy office to work as a sex therapy counselor for high school teenagers in a New York City clinic.

During the past two years, I have employed a registered nurse whose training in addition to a B.S. nursing degree has included special training and experience as patient advocate at a large New York City teaching center. She started as a volunteer and is now employed working a minimum of two full days per week. As a nurse counselor, she deals with the emotional stresses and strains of patients and their families, as well as their interpersonal problems. In addition, she deals with social work aspects of patient care and helps provide nutritional guidance but mostly acts to support patients in a caring, concerned, professional manner, helping to integrate patient care with the various community services available. It is extremely beneficial to the radiation oncologist and technologists to have a person who helps provide aspects of care that are recognized in the day-to-day patient contacts but that the physician and technologists do not have the time to address. The major difficulty in the present situation is still the limited space available and inability of all patient needs and problems to be met by a part-time worker. I still have the problem of funding. At present, the nurse is paid out of income from the practice, and no reimbursement is obtained for her services.

A new office is now under construction. In addition to providing room for new radiation therapy equipment and for better organization of patient flow patterns, space will be provided for the nursing care coordinator on a full-time basis. Rooms will be provided for meditation, imagery, biofeedback, massage, and patient group meetings. A shower will be provided for the use of staff members as a way of encouraging an exercise program that will be initiated for the office staff. A part-time nurse practitioner will be available to coordinate care with respect to meditation, psychologic support, and the like for both staff and patients. The Simonton Method, which involves the use of better coping mechanisms for dealing with stress on a daily basis, will be introduced. This method includes programs of exercise three times per week, encouraging recreation by staff members and patients on a daily basis, and the use of meditation two to three times per day. It is intended to involve the cancer patient in his own care and to help reduce stress among the staff.

The psychological care program will be flexible, adaptable, personalized, and realistic and will be directed to meeting the human needs of patients, their families, and staff; it will be provided during the several weeks that patients are actually undergoing radiation therapy, as well as during follow-up care. The major unresolved problem remains the method of reimbursement for funding these services.

SUMMARY

I have stressed the importance of physician awareness and of psychologic needs of the physician, of the radiation oncology staff, and of the patients and their families. I have indicated the value of personal therapy to aid the physician in integrating these concepts. I would like to emphasize for the future the importance of better training programs involving the incorporation of psychologic and psychosocial theories into the training of physicians and nurses at the medical and nursing school level and in training radiation technologists and radiation oncology residents as they prepare for their professional roles.

Chapter 10

HONESTY IS THE BEST POLICY

A.R. KAGAN, P. LEVITT, THEODORA ARNOLD, AND JEAN HATTEM

When doctors fail to tell a patient with metastatic disease that he is dying, they run the risk of dealing with an angry patient should he discover the truth. Yet, doctors who are candid with their patients invite reactions of a different kind: denial, hysteria, resentment, and rejection of the doctor. As a way of engaging the debate over which is better—telling or not telling—some illustrations from one doctor's (A.R.K.) experiences are presented in this chapter.

In the Regional Radiation Therapy Department of the Southern California Permanente Medical Group, seven patients out of ten have localized cancer, whereas only three out of ten have cancer metastatic to the bone, brain, or other organs. Dying patients are rarely seen. Although many radiation therapists do treat dying patients, I stopped doing so eight years ago because I realized that there comes a time when neither radiation nor chemotherapy can, in certain patients, improve the quality of their lives. Moreover, there are means other than radiation or chemotherapy to alleviate a cancer patient's symptoms.

In my limited experience with terminal cancer patients, I have found that they often ask me perplexing questions about death, dying, and prognosis. Any answer that I give must take into account how much truth the patient can withstand. On the basis of numerous discussions with patients over the past six years (under the direction of T.A.), it has been found that patients are particularly angry with those referring doctors who are evasive and will not give truthful answers to specific questions. As a result of what we have learned from these discussions, our radiation therapists are the first to encourage patients to update their wills and to communicate with wife and family before they become too ill to do these things with the care that they would desire.

A patient for whom radiation therapy holds the promise of cure will be treated for 40 to 180 days and then followed for years, but a terminal patient will be treated sporadically for one to ten days and not be routinely followed. Our aim is to treat terminal patients who need palliation as rapidly as possible. We have found this to be as effective as a prolonged regime. Hence, our intervention in a patient's life is short, and it is easy for us to avoid the patient's questions and to ignore his feelings. Since this is the case, why do we tell the patients the truth? Why do we develop a trusting relationship with him? Why do we risk having the patient turn on us to vent his anger? After all, terminal patients with metastases see many physicians. Why not let the other physicians take the heat?

The answer to these questions is that honesty is the best policy, a statement that has nothing to do with honesty and everything to do with policy. The word *policy* means wise and careful management. Honesty enables us to manage the patient by earning his trust, and we thereby convince him to cooperate fully in his treatment. No doubt an honest appraisal of his illness may cause a patient considerable pain, although often no more than the pain he is caused by lies, evasions, and silences. In any case, the problems arising from a truthful diagnosis, as well as other psychosocial problems, are effectively addressed in our discussions with patients.

Patients, of course, are told different things by different physicians. In general, it has been my experience that most doctors react to terminal patients by giving them less and less information. When the patient insists on a straight answer or asks penetrating questions, the physician more often than not intimidates him with a torrent of technical information and thereby inhibits his ability to cope with his condition. The truth is that doctors are not adequately trained to handle uncomfortable emotional situations; in order to defend themselves, they dismiss the patient's questions as irrelevant or swamp the patient in a morass of medical jargon.

If the radiation therapist believes that he owes the patient the courtesy of gentle candor, the therapist will discover that honesty is the shortest distance between two points. Honesty does away with time-consuming evasion and invites the patient at the outset to disclose his fears and problems. Time spent discussing the truth with a patient is rewarding for both the doctor and the patient. Some case illustrations demonstrate this point.

A sixty-seven-year-old Japanese woman had just been diagnosed as having adenocarcinoma of the entire stomach, omentum, and parts of the peritoneum. I told her that I did not think radiation would be helpful. She asked me about chemotherapy. I advised that if, after the first cycle, the drugs seriously altered the quality of her life, she would be better served by discontinuing chemotherapy. Then she told me that she had three uncles who had died of stomach cancer and that her sister worked with the American Cancer Society. Because of her family's experiences, she was not too enthusiastic about irradiation or chemotherapy and accepted my advice.

The second case concerns a symptomatic doctor with non–oat-cell cancer of the lung that had metastasized to the bone. I told him that I hoped to relieve his symptoms of hemoptysis and pain by irradiating his bronchus and vertebrae but that cure was impossible. I decided we would give him five treatments to each area. He consulted another radiation therapist, who told him that cure was possible but that each site needed thirty treatments. The other radiation therapist telephoned me to complain that my attitude was negative and inexcusable because it conveyed abandonment. The patient's wife was furious with me and urged her husband to see the other radiation therapist, who had indicated that a cure was possible. The patient, however, preferred to remain with me.

A third case concerns a middle-aged, well-to-do lawyer who came to see me because he had been diagnosed with an adenocystic carcinoma of the maxillary sinus. He had just married a very attractive lady who was much younger than he. After a stormy psychological period of denial, the patient agreed to undergo radiation therapy and surgery, which would involve his losing an eye. During radiation therapy the tumor regressed. One week before surgery was scheduled, a new mass distant from the right maxillary sinus was discovered on the upper left gum. The surgeon told the patient that he was incurable and cancelled the surgery. The lawyer reluctantly accepted the surgeon's decision, but not until he had seen other surgeons in the medical community who advised a potpourri of surgical procedures. Our chemotherapist told the patient that there was no effective drug treatment for his disease, but since the cancer was radioresponsive, I treated the new lump.

Not satisfied with our chemotherapist's recommendation, the patient found another chemotherapist. He was given six drugs, hospitalized, and subjected to hyperalimentation and numerous diagnostic tests. The new chemotherapist called me to tell me that over the past few months the tumor had responded well but that unfortunately it always grew back ten days after each drug course. He asked that I give the patient additional radiation. Summoning both the patient and his wife to my office, I told them that the patient's expectation for cure was unrealistic and suggested that they talk to the head of our hospice unit. The patient adamantly refused, but two weeks later, his wife called me to find out more about the services of our hospice and then spoke with its director. Over the next few weeks, I treated the patient for multiple lumps around the eyes and brain. Finally, I reached the point where it was dangerous to add more irradiation. I carefully explained to him the implications of damaging brain, bone, skin, and eye, and gave him a one-week return appointment. He immediately went to see another radiation therapist, who encouraged the patient to enter his care and receive more irradiation. The therapist, as a professional courtesy, informed me of his plan and, at the same time, accused me of abandoning the patient. Is being honest really the same as abandonment?

During my first seven years of medical practice, I worked at institutions that, as a matter of course, revealed to the patient his diagnosis. When I moved to a large private hospital, affiliated with a university, I encountered patients who had not been told the nature of their illnesses or their prognoses. Their referring doctors told them that they had arthritis, or a growth, or an infection, or a precancerous abnormality; that is, they told them anything but the truth. The patients' relatives cooperated in this deception.

As a result, the patients' expectations of what radiotherapy could achieve were unrealistic. The referring doctor had done little or nothing to discourage these expectations and had sometimes covertly encouraged them. Hence some patients with metastatic disease envisioned radiotherapy as a magical cure. In fostering these unrealistic expectations, we administered treatment that I soon came to think of as futile, but when I argued that the treatment did nothing but deplete the patients' strength, my colleagues maintained that it preserved the patients' hope.

These supposedly hopeful patients exhibited, to my mind, a host of psychosocial problems. Ignorant of their diagnosis and understandably suspicious that the truth was being kept from them, they grew angry, came late for appointments or missed them altogether, refused to let the nurse take blood, asked questions that revealed their many fears, and ended by distrusting everyone. From this experience I concluded that patients must be told the truth, lest their fantasies lead them not to pleasant dreams, but to nightmares.

When the referring doctor has lied or remained silent, however, who is to tell the patient the truth? Many radiation therapists think that they are responsible only for treating the patient and not for volunteering any information about his disease. Without information, the patient may expect the treatment to continue long after radiotherapy has ceased to be effective, that is, long after it has ceased to improve the quality of his life. Unless the radiation therapist is willing to tell the patient the truth, he will continue giving therapy, not as a therapeutic measure, but as a means of escaping from the need to tell the patient he is dying.

The radiation therapist must, then, be honest with the patient, but since each patient is different, each must be treated differently. When I discuss cancer with my patients, I begin by assessing the patient's state of mind. Is he frightened or crying? Is he educated or not? Is he willing to talk? Does he know why I am seeing him? What does he consider an acceptable quality of life? If the patient is depressed and needs guidance, I share with him my own views about whether or not treatment is worthwhile. If the patient asks for a prognosis, I give him a reasonable range of possibilities but never a specific answer.

When told the truth about their illnesses, dying patients often choose to forgo treatment, even when their families disapprove of that decision, but it is better for the patient to choose what he thinks best than for the doctor to persuade him to undergo treatment that is expensive and futile. I have seen some dying patients spend as much as 80 percent of their last six months in hospitals or doctors' offices pursuing treatments that are nothing more than a will-o'-the-wisp.

The radiation therapist who tells the patient the truth may be considered by the patient to be cruel, insensitive, and unsympathetic. If the therapist cannot bear this criticism, he can use a group discussion to defuse the patient's anger and to encourage him to come to terms with his illness. In the long run, telling the patient the truth is the best policy because it benefits not only the doctor and his staff but also, most importantly, the patient himself.

BIBLIOGRAPHY

Bok, S. 1978. *Lying: Moral Choices in Public and Private Life.* New York: Pantheon Books.

Cassileth, B.R., D. Volckmar, and R.L. Goodman. 1980. The Effect of Experience on Radiation Therapy Patients' Desire for Information. *International Journal of Radiation Oncology, Biology and Physics, 6:*493-96.

Forester, B.M., D.S. Kornfeld, and J. Fleiss. 1978. Psychiatric Aspects of Radiotherapy. *American Journal of Psychiatry. 135:*8.

Kant, I. 1949. On the Supposed Right to Life from Altruistic Motives. In L.W. Beck, editor and translator, *Critique of Practical Reason.* Chicago: University of Chicago Press.

Litin, E.M., 1960. Should the Cancer Patient Be Told? *Postgraduate Medicine, 28:*470-75.

Rotman, M., L. Rogow, G. DeLeon, and N. Heskel. 1977. Supportive Therapy in Radiation Oncology. *Cancer, 39:*744-50.

Tiger, M.E. 1976. Dying Patients: Less Afraid of the Truth Than We Are. *Medical Economics, 53:*113ff.

Section II

THE RADIATION ONCOLOGY TEAM

PERCEIVED STRESS AND JOB SATISFACTION IN RADIATION THERAPY PROFESSIONALS

WILLIAM J. SOBOTOR AND ROBERT H. SAGERMAN

INTRODUCTION

While much has been written concerning the impact of illness on the patient and the patient's family, little note has been made of the effects of working with cancer patients on the health care provider. Unfortunately, we may have falsely assumed that altruistic motivations can compensate for everyday pressures, thus eliminating environmental or occupational stress in the clinical setting.

Sociologists have defined what goes on within the hospital or clinic as *work* (Glaser and Strauss, 1965; Hall, 1951; Wilson, 1963.) Unpleasant or distasteful as this may seem, the caring for and treatment of ill persons must be organized according to schedule, a specific service rendered, and payment for those services made. Hence, for all practical purposes, medicine, perhaps the most respected of professions, is work and as such is a source of occupational strain. As Moos (1977) states, "Health care professionals enjoy many rewards for their work in terms of intellectual stimulation, social status, and a sense of self-worth based on accomplishment and service to others. However, regular interaction with seriously ill people can be emotionally as well as physically taxing" (p. 367).

73

The hospital, site of most therapeutic endeavors, also adds to the situational stress levels. As Hall (1951) indicated, hospitals are bureaucratic, highly specialized, and conducive to struggles for status and prestige. The social structure of the hospital is highly complex and promotes stress and strain. Administrators regard medical staff as "necessary" mavericks, lest their institution become nothing more than a "hotel for sick people." Nurses as a rule wield immense influence because of sheer numbers and proximity to the job of healing. Other professional groups such as social workers, dietitians, technicians, and pharmacists are in a "no-man's land of prestige" (Wilson, 1963).

Wilson (1963) also described the paradox of modern hospitals. He states, "With the exception of the lowest categories of hospital worker, orderlies and aides, the general principle is that prestige hinges on the extent to which an individual's work entails direct patient care . . ." (p. 72). But "hospital jobs . . . do not foster many paths for smooth progression along a skill hierarchy. Thus, the hospital is a classic illustration of 'blocked mobility'" (p. 75).

The different areas of service within the therapy department may account for varying levels of stress. While the physician is in a decision-making position, the technologist is not. Whereas one prescribes, the other delivers. At the same time, as Newlin and Wellisch (1978) pointed out with the oncology nurse, the technologist "is more constantly and persistently exposed to the emotional vicissitudes and turmoil of the cancer patient and his family."

Hackman and Lawler (1971) described four characteristics that are essential if a task is to provide feelings of achievement, recognition, and personal growth, including: (1) skill variety—the opportunity to utilize a variety of skills, (2) task identity—the opportunity to perform a meaningful part of a project, (3) autonomy—the opportunity to make personal decisions concerning work methods, (4) feedback—the opportunity to learn the effectiveness of one's performance and one's work.

Certainly, both the technologist and the physician share a large degree of skill variety and task identity. Cancer treatment in itself is so diverse that it provides a certain amount of variety. Likewise, few would argue that the various aspects of cancer therapy are not meaningful. Service to others, especially those with life-threatening illnesses, has inherent philosophical value and meaning.

It is in the area of feedback that both levels of health care providers may encounter difficulty. While patients who are cured are a source of positive feedback, thereby reinforcing the meaning in one's work, patients who cannot be cured can serve as negative feedback. This can result in the individual's continual questioning of himself whether or not he is putting forth the best effort. As Dossett (1978) points out, the fear that "one is not working at one's best can be a cause of stress in itself."

Autonomy, the making of decisions concerning one's work, is an essential component of the physician's position. Highly trained and versed in medical science, the physician makes the decision concerning the logistics of patient care. This decision is then transformed into therapeutic plans, and the delivery of the actual treatment is delegated to subordinates.

All staff members, regardless of position, are exposed to a certain amount of stress as a direct result of patient care. While the technologist may be subjected to daily contact with the patient and the family, the physician as the primary caregiver has the ultimate responsibility. In all likelihood, daily front-line pressures on the technologist are equalized by the positional pressures on the physician. Working with cancer patients, in any capacity, is usually a matter of choice, thus suggesting to Hay and Oken (1972) that other areas of care may be less satisfying or even more stressful.

Based on the preceding information, a sample study was designed and implemented to test the following hypotheses:

1. Stress, as a direct result of patient care, is equal across all levels of care provision.
2. Physicians, by virtue of exercising more control over their position, will display greater "job satisfaction."

METHODOLOGY

Subjects

Mail contact was made with twenty-seven radiation therapy department chairpersons in New York State. Names were obtained from the current listing in the American Society of Therapeutic Radiologists roster. Twenty-four responded, agreeing to participate in the study. Based on their estimates of staff participation, 283 forms were mailed. Of these, 141 were returned before the response deadline. Thirty-six of the returned forms were not complete and were eliminated from the analysis. Eight others were eliminated because they were returned by secretaries, aides, and other unqualified personnel. The final sample size was ninety-seven: forty-five physicians and fifty-two technologists.

Instrument Used

The survey form used was designed to tap various aspects of the respondents' perception of their professions. It is based in part on previous forms designed by Brayfield and Rothe (1951), Smith et al. (1969), Rizzo et al. (1970), and Leatt and Schneck (1980).

Correlation among the three sections of the instrument was high in the test items concerning the individual's perception of the profession. No correlation was found between questions dealing with professional duties and responsibilities and perceived stress due to patient care.

RESULTS AND CONCLUSIONS

Tables 11-I and 11-II show results and comparison of significant score differences. In analyzing role stress among nurses, Brief et al. (1979) concluded that it increased with the degree of professional training, with baccalaureate degree nurses experiencing the greatest stress. In the sample, contrary results were obtained with respondents' job satisfaction. Initial analysis shows physicians scoring highest on satisfaction scales, technologists with baccalaureate and associate degrees next highest, and technologists with only radiation therapy training scoring lowest.

A closer examination of the data revealed several interesting results. Data concerning overall job satisfaction show a significant difference between staff radiation therapists and female technologists ($\alpha = .01$) and staff radiation therapists and male technologists with a degree and with only radiation therapy training ($\alpha = .01$).

Overall stress levels were nonsignificant with two exceptions.

Table 11-I
MEAN SCORES OF GROUPS ON VARIOUS SUBSETS OF TEST ITEMS

		Perception of Profession	Duties & Responsibilities	Patient Care Stress
	Physician (Staff)	15.21	8.06	39.27
	Physician (Resident)	12.75	5.16	35.83
	♀ Technologist	10.60	2.46	29.32
	♂ Technologist	5.00	-3.00	32.75
AAS BS BA	♀ Technologist	14.00	4.80	34.20
	♂ Technologist	6.33	1.66	32.77

Table 11-II
SUMMARY OF SIGNIFICANT SCORE DIFFERENCE RESULTS

Staff Radiation Therapist Versus		Perception of Profession	Duties & Responsibilities	Patient Care Stress
	Physician (Resident)	NS	.05	NS
	♀ Technologist	.01	.001	.0001
	♂ Technologist	.01	.0001	.05
AAS BS BA	♀ Technologist	NS	.02	NS
	♂ Technologist	.01	.0001	NS

Staff therapists showed less stress than female technologists ($\overline{\alpha}$ = .0001) and male technologists with either an associate or baccalaureate degree (α = .05).

In the respondents' perception of the duties and responsibilities of their professions, all comparisons with staff therapists showed significant differences and overall job satisfaction as follows: therapy residents (α = .05), female technologists (α = .001), female technologists with associate or baccalaureate degree (α = .02), male technologists with associate or baccalaureate degree (α = .0001), and male technologists (α = .0001).

Evidently, there is an interaction between educational level and sex that takes place in radiation therapy professionals' perception of their job satisfaction.

Being exploratory in nature, this study suffers several deficits. Care must be exercised before attempting to generalize and apply these findings to training and hiring practices.

No control was possible for the effect of hospital type or size. Miller (1976), for example, found distinct, significant differences when analyzing nurse role stress as a function of different hospital environments. Likewise, Snoek (1966) found organizational size to be directly related to tension levels among various members of the organizations.

At the same time, no effort was made to obtain information concerning respondents' geographic location or salary levels. Perhaps some of the results could be modified in a future study, which would include control for location and salary.

Activity levels of the various departments were likewise unknown. It is impossible to identify what portion of the findings is solely due to excessive patient loads and insufficient staffing.

Nevertheless, some interesting conclusions can be drawn from the project. Goode (1960) states that most jobs fall into a rather ambiguous category wherein there exist inconsistencies or contradictory expectations. The staff therapist, of all respondent groups, has the most consistent role expectations. His patients expect optimal care; colleagues expect ethical and professional behavior; he himself expects to apply himself with utmost zeal. He has reached the ultimate on the educational ladder; all subsequent learning is to make him "more expert." Decisions are made by him, and these are transferred into therapeutic prescriptions and passed down to others to deliver. It may well be that the staff therapist's position is generally viewed by those occupying that position as comprising the four essential characteristics described earlier by Hackman and Lawler (1971).

Compared with this position, the status of the resident physician is less concrete. He is still in a definitive learning process. Experience at this level is intended to mold him into a true professional. Duties and responsibilities are less clear, less formally structured. Any decision that is made is to be approved by superiors before implementation. These restrictions could partially account for decreased job satisfaction.

Most interesting are the findings among the technologists. Among females, those technologists with only technical training evidenced increased perceived stress levels when compared with females with advanced education. Several factors may be operating here, including the possibility that those with more education are in supervisory positions, spend more time in educating students, and may also have more opportunity for continuing education. At the same time, it may well be that the more educated female technologist perceives herself as a true professional, an integral member of a treatment team. The less educated female may view herself as less involved in the team approach. Perhaps this is a replication of Feldman's (1976) finding that better educated nurses place more emphasis on total patient care—both physical and emotional—thereby deriving more satisfaction from their profession.

Male technologist respondents provoke much speculation concerning their responses. While both the technically trained and the degree groups scored nearly the same on perceived stress, there were widely discrepant results in their job satisfaction scores. Both groups scored lowest on job satisfaction, regardless of educational level. Several areas need to be explored here. Is this the residual of a cultural bias that continues to emphasize the feminine aspects of the health care profession? In other words, is this the same reverse sex discrimination that existed in the nursing profession? Does the male feel less of a sense of job identity or integrity than his female counterpart? Or is it because males are supposed to achieve, and radiation therapy offers little room for personal advancement beyond a certain level? As Wilensky (1964) argued, it may well be that the male technologist has difficulty fitting into the hierarchical scheme of medicine and is less content to accept the delegation of work such a status system entails.

The findings in this project should engender future research. Most technologists with degree educations indicated their education and abilities were not always maximally utilized, corroborating earlier findings of Brief et al. (1979) when investigating registered nurses. This may be the result of the emphasis on professionalization. As Corwin (1961) found in his nurse's study, this project may be tapping several different and divergent conceptions of the technologist role.

Since almost all subgroup stress scores were nonsignificant, one is tempted to conclude that patient care is not the main factor in job satisfaction. Subgroups, when responding to specific patient-care issues, scored relatively equally. The only major areas of difference were noted in questions dealing with one's own perception of one's profession and with duties and responsibilities. Stress, then, is not seen as an integral part of patient care. Rather, it is seen as directly related to one's sense of job identity or integrity. All respondent subgroups appear equally capable of coping with the patient care aspects of their position. It appears that the critical element in determining one's job satisfaction is not the patient-provider relationship but the sex of the care provider and his place in the care-providing hierarchy.

REFERENCES

Brayfield, A.H. and H. F. Rothe. 1951. An Index of Job Satisfaction. *Journal of Applied Psychology, 35(5):*307-11.

Brief, A.P., M.V. Sell, R.J. Aldag, and N. Melone. 1979. Anticipatory Socialization and Role Stress Among Registered Nurses. *Journal of Health and Social Behavior, 20:*161-66.

Corwin, R.G. 1961. Role Conception and Career Aspiration: A Study of Identity in Nursing. *Sociological Quarterly, 2:* 69-86.

Dossett, S.M. 1978. Nursing Staff in High Dependency Areas. *Nursing Times,* May 25, 888-89.

Feldman, D.C. 1976. A Contingency Theory of Socialization. *Administrative Science Quarterly, 21:*433-52.

Glaser, B. and A.L. Strauss. 1965. *Awareness of Dying: A Study of Social Interaction.* New York: Macmillan.

Goode, W.J. 1960. A Theory of Role Strain. *American Sociological Review,* 25:483-96.

Hackman, J.R. and E.E. Lawler. 1971. Employee Reactions to Job Characteristics. *Applied Psychology, 55(3):*259-86.

Hall, O. 1951. Sociological Research in the Field of Medicine: Progress and Prospects. *American Sociological Review, 16:* 639-44.

Hay, D. and D. Oken. 1972. The Psychological Stresses of Intensive Care Unit Nursing. *Psychosomatic Medicine, 34(2):*109.

Leatt, P. and R. Schneck. 1980. Differences in Stress Perceived by Headnurses Across Nursing Specialties in Hospitals. *Journal of Advanced Nursing, 5:* 31-46.

Miller, G.A. 1976. Patient Knowledge and Nurse Role Strain in Three Hospital Settings. *Medical Care, 14(8):*662-73.

Moos, R.H., ed. 1977. *Coping with Physical Illness.* New York: Plenum Medical Book Company.

Newlin, N.J. and D.K. Wellisch. 1978. The Oncology Nurse: Life on an Emotional Roller Coaster. *Cancer Nursing,* December, 447-49.

Rizzo, J.R., R.J. House, and S.I. Lirtzman. 1970. Role Conflict and Ambiguity in Complex Organizations. *Administrative Science Quarterly, 15:*150-63.

Smith, P.C., L.M. Kendall, and C.L. Hulin. 1969. *The Measurement of Satisfaction in Work and Retirement.* Chicago, Rand McNally and Company.

Snoek, J.D. 1966. Role Strain in Diversified Role Sets. *The American Journal of Sociology, 71(4):*363-72.

Wilensky, H.L. 1964. The Professionalization of Everyone? *The American Journal of Sociology, 70 (2):*137-58.

Wilson, R.N. 1963. The Social Structure of a General Hospital. *Annals of the American Academy of Political and Social Science, 346:*67-76.

Chapter 12

THE IMPACT OF RADIATION ONCOLOGY ON THE STAFF

R USHDY A BADIR

THE RADIATION ONCOLOGIST

T he image of a radiation oncologist as health care provider is modeled not only by the obvious factors such as the medical background and personality characteristics but also by the specific circumstances of that specialty. Several factors contribute to the formation of the ultimate image and will be discussed.

Issues of Survival, or the Image of Cancer

"Do you feel depressed dealing with cancer patients all the time?" This is an invariable question that a stranger asks in trying to start a conversation with a radiation oncologist (or radiation technologist) after knowing the nature of his work. Subconsciously, when talking about cancer, the healthy individual divides people into (1) dying and (2) others and places the cancer patient in the first category. This reaction toward cancer patients is part of the psychology of the lay persons in dealing with a radiation oncologist. The impact on the radiation oncologist of dealing with cancer patients with fatal or potentially curable disease is perhaps no different from that of other diseases and other physicians. In the 1960s and before, chemotherapy played a far smaller role for the cancer patient than it plays now; therefore, at that time the radiation therapist represented practically the final stage of referral of the cancer patient for nonsurgical treatment. This became more apparent when the radiation therapist actually supervised the chemotherapy, as was the case in Britain and some other countries. At the present time, the radiation oncologist sees fewer dying cancer patients, who are now seen more often by the chemotherapists. However, the radiation oncologists who practiced in the 1960s or earlier are aware of the unspoken feeling among medical professionals that radiation therapy served as a sort of undertaker of the medical profession. Although radiation therapy has cured many cancers, the image of the radiation therapy patient as the terminal cancer patient has been a dominant one. Deficiencies in teaching the potentials of radiation therapy to undergraduate medical students helped to mask the curing potentials of radiation therapy and left only a poor image. At the present time, a good part of that image persists despite the fact that terminal patients are now referred, to a large extent, to the chemotherapist rather than to the radiation oncologist. Only education of other specialties can avoid this situation, but opportunities for such education are difficult to find in either pre- or postgraduate stages.

The Rad

Contrary to the unit used in medications, which is mainly the gram, the radiation therapist uses a unit not used by any other physician for prescriptions, that is, the rad. As a result, there is classification of the physicians into gram-users, and these are the majority, and rad-users, who are the minority. Some have referred to gram-users as the "real doctors," especially since most radiation oncologists do not have bed assignments. This feeling is noticeable among the younger generations who had been practicing "traditional" medicine shortly before specialization in therapeutic radiology.

The Irreversible Effect of the Rad

Not only is the unit of radiation different from the unit of chemical medications, but also the effect of each is different.

Chemicals used as medications can be excreted, detoxified, or metabolized with ultimate elimination of their effect. Once a dose of radiation is given, however, its biological effect usually cannot be erased and is cumulative.

This irreversible effect of the rad has an impact on its deliverers. A radiation oncologist is and should be a meticulous observer of the therapy delivery system. This attitude entails a nonpermissive execution of treatment. In a large institution, a domineering image of the supervisors may be created. Such supervisors may be physicians, technologists, or physicists. Those working in the field with clear understanding of the requirements of the specialty accept and expect a tight routine. It is obvious that a lot of the interpretation of the final image depends on the interpreter. Some describe this as "good and accurate," and others describe it as "dictatorial." The radiation oncologist, especially the chief of the service, reaps the ultimate result of the interpretation. There is no doubt that this is a stressful situation for the radiation oncologist and the rest of his staff.

Geographical Location within a Building

Because of the heavy shielding needed for the therapeutic ionizing radiation, radiation therapy departments are built in the lowest level of a building, usually the basement. Location in the basement may be associated with unsightly surroundings, such as proximity to workships, storage area, freight area, and so forth, which are usually gloomy and depressing. Of all the stressful factors associated with radiation therapy, perhaps location is the worst. At the present time, there is a trend to build new departments that avoid that image. Although the progress is consistent, it is slow because of the incurred expenses and lack of space in many instances.

Expensive Equipment

Of all the expenses incurred in the management of human cancer in the United States, radiotherapy costs only about 3 percent of the total amount (400,000 cancer patients annually costing $30 billion, of which $1 billion is for radiotherapy

[Powers, n.d.]). Considering the overall curative and palliative value of radiotherapy, it is a relatively cheap modality of treatment; therefore, capital expenditure is well justified. Unfortunately, in practical life, it is difficult to raise funds for radiotherapy because of the high initial expenses. Therefore, the radiation oncologist in most instances works under strenuous conditions with minimal appropriations for modernizing the capital equipment. Old cobalt units, lack of simulators, lack of planning computers, and lack of space are well-known circumstances in many radiation oncology centers all over the world. Struggle with the administration for basic requirements is a constant in the life of a practicing radiotherapist. The question of whether to have two centers in two hospitals in the same area or only one larger center has been a source of strain and stress to radiotherapists in so many locations that it seems to be a rule of the specialty. Such circumstances create an unstable, stressful atmosphere.

The Department of Radiology, Section of Radiotherapy

The status of radiation oncology as a section of the department of radiology has probably retarded the development of therapeutic radiology in the United States (Abadir, 1977). Fortunately, in the past few years, separation of radiation oncology into an independent department is noted in several centers, but the rate of separation is not fast enough. The dependence of radiation therapy on diagnostic radiology is due to the historical development of radiotherapy; it was delivered by diagnostic radiologists. At that time, the dependence was expected, but it continued after radiotherapy separated as a discipline and the specialist became an oncologist, distinctly different from a diagnostic radiologist. The interests of therapeutic radiology may conflict with those of diagnostic radiology or may not be fully conceived by diagnostic radiologists acting as chairmen of a combined department.

Impact of Medical Oncology on Radiation Oncology

The interaction of the surgeon with the radiation oncologist is traditional, since radiation was used for the therapy of cancer.

Occasionally, competition between the surgeon and the radiation oncologist evolves, but this is often healthy and complementary.

Medical oncology grew very fast in the 1970s and had to interact more and more with radiation oncology. The presence of a relatively large number of chemotherapists working in the wards close to the cancer patients and their referring physicians and residents under the label of *"the* oncologist" created a situation in which the radiation oncologist is now being displaced by the medical oncologist from the first line of referral. Often, cases are referred for radiation therapy because the chemotherapist so advised. Cases are occasionally referred for radiation therapy rather than for the opinion of the radiation oncologist.

Radiation oncologists are fully aware of and frustrated by this situation. Del Regato and Pittman (1980) have rightly expressed that notion in the field of education by describing the ubiquitous medical oncologists' acquiring positions of influence, with medical students exposed disproportionately to total management of cancer by drugs without proper information about the irreplaceable role of radiotherapy.

Worse than the placement of radiotherapy under the department of diagnostic radiology is the incorporation of radiation oncology into a department of oncology including medical oncology. This causes radiation oncology not only to lose fiscal independence but also to lose medical independence (Moss, 1976). Fortunately, this trend seems to be less vigorous now than five years ago.

Cure by Radiation

Radiation can achieve cure of cancer without mutilation. This strength of the specialty ironically led to a controversial result for the radiation oncologist. Being reassured by the curative ability of the modality, both surgeons and radiation oncologists have been less active in competing for research money; however, chemotherapy, which is mainly a palliative modality, successfully competed for and received the largest proportion of clinical research funds. The justification for this is that chemotherapy is a developing modality and confusing to use. The end result has been that radiation oncologists with their small numbers and minimal research funds are confronted by medical oncologists with their larger numbers and the strength of abundant research funds.

Relative Number of Specialists

The number of physicians working in radiation oncology is relatively small. Typically, many radiotherapy centers are staffed by only two members: One is chief, and the other is his associate. Such a situation creates its effect on the physicians working in the field. A major effect is the lack of noise in committees of administrative influence. This situation of numerical minority leads to difficulty in vital issues such as funding, curricula, and so forth. The result in excessive frustration.

Opportunities for Private Practice

The opportunities for private practice in radiation oncology are remarkably fewer than those in other specialties. The reason for this is the high initial expense of equipment as well as the limited patient resources within an area where there is often one or more major hospital-based center. Most radiation oncologists are therefore captive audiences to hospital appointments with their limitations.

A frustrating limitation in hospital appointments is that radiation oncologists often cannot get constructive ideas for departmental planning implemented because various authorities such as the administrator and the dean cannot be convinced. The rest of the story repeats itself, and eventually the center is abandoned by radiotherapists, with further deterioration of the service. The administration then moves to adopt all or some of the ideas for which the previous radiation oncologists had been calling. This may happen in departments other than radiotherapy, but undoubtedly it happens on a much larger scale in radiation oncology because of the large amount of capital involved. In other disciplines, private practice is a safety valve for frustration, but that opportunity does not lend itself readily to a radiation oncologist.

THE RADIATION THERAPY TECHNOLOGIST

Many of the factors that affect radiation oncologists affect the technologist as well. Dealing with terminal illness is a major factor coloring the profession. It is fortunate that, in general, radiotherapy technologists have good understanding of their role in cancer, both the curable and the incurable. The location of the department in the basement is as depressing to the technologists as it is to the physicians. Maintaining meticulous observation of precise treatment is a stress that the radiation technologist shares with the physician. The lack of space and slow change of equipment impede the technologist also. Other problems are more specific to the technologist.

Treatment Is Given, Not Taken—Shortage of Technologists

Contrary to medications that can be taken by the patient, radiation treatment must be given and cannot be self-administered, and the technologist is the one who gives the treatment. The technologist is, therefore, the umbilical cord of the provision of health care in radiation therapy.

The total dependence on the technologist for delivery of therapy has its negative effects. A feeling of self-importance is a pronounced consequence. If that feeling is magnified in the technologist's mind, he may either be increasingly giving or increasingly demanding. The giving technologist is the one who realizes that he deals with a life-threatening disease and gives the needed and expected support. A demanding technologist is the one who takes advantage of the desperate need for technologists and "spoils" himself with the belief that he cannot be replaced. Both the giving and the demanding technologists are seen in practical life, and both aspects may be present in the same person.

Technologist-Patient Relationship

The feelings and expectations of a patient toward a technologist are different from those directed toward a physician. The patient expects more sympathetic talk from the technologist than from the physician. The technologist realizes this and feels the same way. Unfortunately, in "standard" working conditions the situation is rather rushed, with time for actual delivery of treatment but little time for comforting, friendly talk with the patient. The result is that both the patient and the technologist may be frustrated by the deficiency.

The technologist falls between a doctor demanding perfection and a patient demanding attention. Because of this, technologists may develop feelings of guilt. Alternatively, with the pressure of work a technologist may develop a feeling of hostility toward a patient or some patients. This situation may be improved by employing a sufficient number of technologists, but this is not feasible at the present time due to a nationwide shortage.

The patient also is given information by the referring physician or members of his team such as residents or medical students. There is a serious deficiency in knowledge about radiation among "nonradiation" doctors, who may believe that much harm and many side effects can be attributed to radiation therapy. This apprehension is cultivated in the patient, who relates his feelings more readily to the technologist than to the radiation oncologist. The radiation technologist is frustrated with a situation in which inaccurate or incorrect, frightening information is passed to a patient about the radiation that the technologist is giving for the patient's benefit.

Technologist-Doctor Relationship

The cancer patient load referred to radiotherapy is usually demanding, with the pressure put on the radiation oncologist. Ultimately, this load is placed on the shoulders of the technologist. The overall picture appears to be one in which a pressed doctor pushes a technologist to get the work accomplished. Most technologists are understanding and obliging and try their best to get the maximum work done. However, the day's work usually passes as a routine; the work gets done with goodwill and cooperation from technologists who ultimately may be disappointed that they did not receive appreciation for what they did. This is particularly frustrating because mistakes are not tolerated in radiation therapy and good work is not routinely praised.

Technologist-Technologist Relationship

It is normal for the aim of work to be earning a salary. However, professional accomplishment seems to dominate work image in many instances. The experienced senior technologist gets well oriented toward the professional aspects of work, while the young technologist with limited experience may seem to work for the money with little more concern for the profession than what is necessary to hold a job. This negative attitude toward professional performance may draw criticism and concern by supervisory or senior technologists.

Routine monotonous working conditions do not offer a stimulating environment, nor does the shortage of funds for an adequate number of professional meetings help. Junior technologists, therefore, may tend to blame senior colleagues partially for the shortcomings. Change of jobs is a frequent outlet, especially since positions may be available in most centers.

SUMMARY

Radiation oncology as a profession places stress on the physicians and technologists working in that field. The major stressors are the geographical locations of the treatment sites, the slow upgrading of equipment or the facility, the lack of tolerance of mistakes, the ignorance of the full scope of radiation oncology among other medical specialties, and the potentially fatal nature of the diseases being treated. The outcome is generally frustration, and the outlet is frequently a change of jobs.

REFERENCES

Abadir, R. 1977. Separate Radiotherapy Oncology Department. *International Journal of Radiation Oncology, Biology, and Physics*, 2:1045-46.

Del Regato, J.A. and D.D. Pittman. 1980. The Training of Radiotherapists in the United States. *Internal Journal of Radiation Oncology, Biology, and Physics*, 6:1705-10.

Moss, W.T. 1976. Out of the Frying Pan Into the Fire? *Radiology, 118*:741.

Powers, W. n.d. Personal communication.

Chapter 13

GOOD PATIENTS AND BAD PATIENTS
A Sociologist Looks at Radiation Therapy Staff
TRISH LITTMAN

This study examines the ways work-related tensions were managed by different levels of staff in a radiotherapy department and the consequences of strategies developed by staff to maximize occupational satisfactions and minimize the negative aspects of their daily work activities. Radiation oncology, while primarily consultative and clinical, poses problems of caring and curing similar to those found in other medical specialties, such as psychiatry, postoperative surgical intensive-care units, and chronic care facilities. In common with these specialties, radiotherapy involves a potentially high degree of doubt and frustration about the effectiveness of ministrations or interventions. Given the nature of this specialty and the current limitations of scientific knowledge and therapeutic technology, tensions are likely to develop between the demands of one's work and the needs of the patients. How the radiation therapists, nursing staff, and radiation therapy technicians balanced those tensions significantly affected their relations with each other and with patients.

Nearly all of the thirty members of the radiation therapy staff at one teaching hospital were interviewed. A key question was to define "good and bad patients." In brief, patients were compositely evaluated as "good" when they reciprocally communicated, positively cooperated, made appropriate demands, looked well, were curable, and expressed gratitude for the care they received. The caring staff felt their work was effective with such patients.

Patients were evaluated as "bad" when they made excessive or insatiable demands, were uncooperative or ungrateful, looked sick or had an unesthetic appearance, were incurable, or became worse in spite of all ministrations. The caring staff felt their efforts were insignificant or depreciated by such patients.

Each staff level had it particular set of these definitions, specialized ministrations or work tasks, and corresponding degree of freedom to seek work satisfactions. The radiotherapists, nurses, nurse's assistants, and radiation therapy technicians consistently emphasized the sustaining importance of their relationships with patients as well as with colleagues. Through these kinds of meaningful associations, the work-related tensions were managed. While these relationships were theoretically available to all staff, opportunities for their selective cultivation were differentially distributed. The physicians enjoyed the greatest number of options for shielding themselves from excessive doubt and frustration; the nursing staff were less free but still had room to pursue personal interests; the radiation therapy technicians had the least number of choices.

FINDINGS AND DISCUSSION

Radiation Therapists

How the physicians viewed their particular work role, especially the subjective meanings of caring for patients, determined the kinds of patients and relationships that would be sought. The radiation therapists, including the residents, associated "good patients" with engaging personalities and reciprocal communication, intellectually or technically challenging diseases, and potentially curable cancers without complications or refractory problems. Medically, the "good patients" were linked by the physicians with primary breast tumors, Hodgkin's disease, certain gynecologic cancers of ovaries and cervix, and, to a lesser extent, lymphomas and some leukemias. The five-year survival rates for these diseases are generally high. All radiotherapists maintained a significant percentage of these "good patients" in their case loads, with the following consequences.

First, the favorable survival rates were personally gratifying ("I,

Dr. Doe, saved this patient's life.") and professionally satisfying ("Radiation therapy cured these patients.") Second, the patients were pleased and expressed their appreciation and even awe. Third, within the department, subspecialization brought recognition of an implied expertise, as well as the territory it covered. By staking out a certain type or stage of disease, the radiotherapist unwittingly introduced some competition and even disgruntlement into daily relations with colleagues. Finally, outside the department, respect given by other physicians for the implied expertise of subspecialization represented a personalized projection of the high survival rates onto the specific radiotherapist. ("Dr. Doe is that department's special Hodgkin's person.") Since the referring physician and the radiotherapist probably shared overlapping medical definitions of "good patients," their reputations were mutually reinforcing with their treatment of these particular diseases. In this way, the radiotherapists were able to attract consultations for certain types or stages of disease and thus could assure themselves an acceptable proportion of "good patients."

The physicians viewed as "bad" those patients who were unesthetic, incurable, or uncommunicative. Medically, they linked these patients with advanced, recurrent, metastatic, or fungating diseases beyond the reaches of their radically curative interventions. Moreover, the radiotherapists' atitudes toward palliation were ambivalent at best and commonly apologetic. One doctor remarked, "As medical care, it's noble, but it won't get you a Nobel." Although palliation and "bad patients" were not necessarily synonymous, they were not exciting either.

The radiotherapists' high status in the department permitted them multiple avenues for forming sustaining relationships with patients and other physicians, both within and outside the department. In response to their working definitions of "good and bad patients," these physicians could select certain types and stages of disease ("good cancers") in which to subspecialize, use residents to perform certain unpleasant or undesirable tasks, design their own individualized programs combining basic research with clinical practice, or elect certain administrative positions, such as program development. This array made them feel effective, while it also enhanced relationships and shielded them from the negative aspects of their daily work. However, these choices also reinforced the physicians' independence. With their considerable freedom came a dual separation. The options available to the physicians not only hindered the development of fellow-feeling among them as a group but also protected them from prolonged contact with "bad patients." Separation and avoidance were firmly established on the physicians' level, among themselves and with incurable or otherwise objectionable patients.

Nursing Staff

The nurses and nurse's assistants considered esthetics, cure rates, and stage of disease less important than a patient's willingness to participate in a working relationship. For them, nursing meant caring and communicating. This group focused their multifunctional ministrations on any needs or aspects of daily living that the patient and they identified. A patient who was technically challenging or personally responsive and who made a mutually desirable improvement, even a very small gain, was viewed as "good." Patients with overly demanding and inconsiderate personalities were viewed as "bad." Their insensitivity to others and their exclusive self-absorption impeded effective communication and thus restricted the efficacy of nursing staff's work.

Nursing staff enjoyed a moderate amount of freedom and flexibility in sustaining satisfying relationships among themselves and with other members of the department, as well as with patients. Yet, without an adequate number of staff, strong leadership, and clear guidelines for their work roles and tasks, they lacked unifying organization. They expressed frustration, claiming they were not accorded recognition and respect, particularly by physicians. How these nurses and nurse's assistants individually defined the particular tasks and meanings of their roles largely determined the extent to which occupational satisfactions were attainable. In addition, by taking on administrative or quasi-managerial tasks, such as associating with national clinical research protocols, the nurses could select some of the types of disease they would care for and thus pursue areas of personal interest. Such latitude provided opportunities for creative, gratifying interventions but restricted their ministrations to a circumscribed number of "good patients." Nursing staff lacked cohesion and were somewhat dissociated from the other staff.

Radiation Therapy Technicians

The technicians viewed as "good" those patients who were willing and easy to communicate with. That definition encompassed patient personality, mobility, and the appointment schedule. Without excessive demands, the treatment and the interaction between technician and patient could proceed smoothly. "Bad patients" were disagreeable or nonambulatory. They took time from other scheduled patients by demanding their personal needs be met and required extra assistance in being set up for treatment. Patients who were immobile or uncommunicative because of illness (such as paralysis or tracheotomy) were not necessarily "bad," however. Additional help significantly reduced the quality and quantity of one-on-one interaction. Thus, the relentlessness of time and patient census intensified an already rigorous job.

The demanding work conditions were even more stressful because the technicians served as "flak-catchers" from patients and other staff, particularly physicians. Patients who were physically difficult to treat or who had insatiably demanding personalities slowed down the technicians' fast rhythm. Sometimes a machine would break down for several days. Often, patients had to wait a long time to be treated. They usually vented their anger on the technicians or occasionally complained directly to the radiotherapist. Either way, visibility and availability turned the technicians into convenient targets of patient and staff frustration.

In addition to delays, other aspects of daily work further taxed the technicians. First, under duress, their routine tasks threatened to turn into assembly line work, thus removing a major source of job satisfaction. Every technician cited intense, meaningful interaction with patients as their main compensation for occupational negatives. Several compared this benefit with the depersonalized atmosphere they attributed to their work in diagnostic radiology.

Second, the technicians labored under the burden of "error by a hair." Not only did they have to manage the treatment process speedily, they also had to re-create for each patient, each day on treatment, a 100 percent accurate technical setup. Although quality control had eased this burden somewhat, administrative rules to correct that situation often lacked systematic follow-through and thus added more rancor and frustration.

The technicians doubly bore the brunt of technical errors. They expressed feelings of guilt, holding themselves personally responsible for any slight oversights or minor inaccuracies that may have caused their patients additional discomfort or anguish. Also, the technicians were held accountable by the radiotherapists, who relied on them to execute their treatment directives. These physicians were generally regarded as unappreciative or insensitive to the stresses of the technicians' job. Yet, the technicians often displayed the same lack of insight into the dilemmas of the physicians' work situation as they claimed was directed at theirs.

Finally, the technicians' typical daily tasks contributed to their occupational rigors. For example, they were trained to perform the same skills, and in this way all worked interchangeably. Subspecialization was not available to them, unless they wanted to end patient interaction (their saving grace) and work in dosimetry and physics. Administrative positions were already filled and were foreclosed to them. Two technicians rotated as floaters, helping out wherever necessary. These roles did not particularly relieve stress but often increased it and severely curtailed continuity of patient contact. So, the technicians' daily round of activities contributed significantly to the tension between the demands of their work and the needs of the patients.

The technicians thus had the least freedom to protect themselves from negative aspects of their work. They received the lowest financial, status, and power rewards, yet exhibited extraordinarily high degrees of solidarity, mutual support, and resilience under work conditions of sustained tension and stress. Having so few choices, they were forced to form their own camaraderie. Their occupation and status constraints enabled them to achieve a significant group spirit that was noticeably absent for the other staff levels. Although their camaraderie was compensatory, it limited their sustaining relations to themselves and patients and did not foster sympathetic understanding of the dilemmas facing nursing staff and radiotherapists.

CONCLUSIONS

In this study, perceptions of occupational roles and satisfactions were contained in the three sets of definitions for "good patients." Prolonged contact with these patients provided a sense that one's interventions were effective and worthwhile. Mutual and sympathetic understandings were shared in reciprocal relationships with patients and colleagues. On the other hand, the definitions of "bad patients" revealed the tension between work demands and patient needs characteristic of each staff level.

Strategies that enhanced sustaining relationships depended on one's position in the department. To varying degrees, the existing alternatives protected the physicians, nursing staff, and technicians from extensive, unrelieved, and frustrating contact with "bad patients." However, those strategies not only encouraged isolation by avoiding or withdrawing emotional investment from certain patients, they also prevented appreciation of the tasks and dilemmas of other staff.

In radiation oncology, the management of work-related tension can be ultimately demoralizing. Regardless of political and administrative considerations that were not included in this study, separation was found to be endemic in this department, reaching everyone and affecting all relationships. "Bad patients" were penalized for their diseases or for their personality defects. Hope, enthusiasm, and support were largely withheld from them. They thus suffered the greatest losses.

Since the data were restricted to one location, caution must be exercised in generalizing from the findings. However, by formulating the problem broadly, it was hoped the study could be replicated in other radiation therapy departments as well as in similar occupational settings, within medicine and elsewhere, and that the insights gained in this investigation would have comparative relevance and wider application.

SHARED CONTROL IN THE PRACTICE OF RADIATION ONCOLOGY
Theoretical Framework

NINA H. DIAMOND, RICHARD WHITTINGTON, PHILIP LICHTENBERG, AND MOHAMMED MOHIUDDIN

The position of members of the radiation oncology team as consultants in the cancer care system is inherently conflictual. While the explicit goal of this system is provision of comprehensive coordinated care for the patient, the practical reality is often fragmentation of care on all levels. The clinical radiation oncology team consists of the radiation oncologist, the radiation technologist, the nurse, and the social worker. Since this team is rarely in a position of total system leadership, this limits its power in determining treatment outcome. The exclusionary behaviors sometimes exhibited by fellow oncology colleagues serve to exaggerate the team's sense of limited power and interfere with the unity of the system as a whole, with the care of the patients, and with the effectiveness of the team.

The focus of this chapter is on team members' perceived inadequacy of power in the cancer care system as an issue affecting optimal treatment outcome and patient/staff satisfaction. A review of the literature demonstrates that with respect to the issues of power and control, there are distinct sets of problems that confront patients and that these very issues affect and apply to the therapeutic team as well. Attempted solutions have only partially addressed the problems. Such attempts have focused on change, both in the psychological status of patients, caregivers, and systems and in the social status of these groups. Although these efforts have achieved some success, they have failed in the ultimate goal of providing an efficient, effective, and satisfying treatment system.

This chapter proposes alternative conceptualizations of both issues and solutions that involve redefinition of organizational patterns. Optimal satisfaction and effectiveness can be achieved only when all participants in the process share control and power in a democratic, as opposed to an authoritarian, fashion. The radiation oncology team must be reorganized as a subsystem of membership groups, each of whom has vested interests in the treatment outcome, as well as unique areas of expertise. Each group must be allowed to engage in decision making and planning to the degree to which its expertise permits. This not only will result in shared power, control, responsibility, and accountability but will have broader effects for the patient and in the cancer care system at large.

IDENTIFIED ISSUES

Several sets of issues have repeatedly emerged as critical problem areas in a primarily patient-focused literature. In this chapter they are identified as issues of *control, power, affective stances,* and *communication patterns.* It is apparent that for each patient problem, there exists a matching problem for staff. This is not surprising, since both patients and caregivers are embedded in the same system, both psychologically and socially. Thus, the system's structural limitations can compound the limitations of its participants (Kleiman et al., 1977), just as the individual's psychological framework can reinforce the weaknesses of the system. When individuals have fears about death, they easily support a system that promotes the denial of death.

Underlying all other issues is the fundamental issue of perceived internal and external *control* of self and others (Bahnson, 1975; Enelow, 1976; Nelson et al., 1978; Sadowski et al., 1978; Schmale, 1976). This is a central issue because the very nature of this work concerns that which we perceive as the ultimate loss of control—death. For patients, fear of loss of control is a major concern, from which emanate their attempts to cope as cancer patients and with medical staff. Patients express uncertainty about the nature and outcome of treatment (Prior, 1976), projection of unrealistic feelings and expectations upon caregivers (Bahnson, 1975; Konior and Levine, 1975; Krant and Johnston, 1977), fear of abandonment (Konior and Levine, 1975; Krant, 1976), vacillations between intense anger and depression (Craig and Abeloff, 1974; Plumb and Holland, 1977), increased manifestations of dependency (Holland, 1977), and attribution of omnipotence to the radiation oncology team (Koocher, 1979; Krant, 1976; McIntosh, 1974; Schnaper, 1977; Schulz and Aderman, 1976). These are but a few examples of anticipated or actual loss of control. Because radiation staff share the same fear of death and professionally they equate death of patients with diminution or lack of control on their part, they resonate with their patient's concerns. They grasp at the controls they do have and often act out inaccurate, inappropriate, and inadequate forms of pseudocontrol (Baider, 1975). This appears in behaviors that include attempts solely and/or heroically to control treatment and to avoid patient/staff interactions that challenge this false sense of potency. The interplay of mutual concerns around control results in erection of psychological barriers to effective medical and psychosocial intervention and in reinforcement of social systems that promote an authoritarian hierarchy, which is characterized by unilateral decision making downward. The inevitable by-product of organizing in this fashion is increased anger, desperation, and isolation at the time when staff most need a balanced control system, that is, when treatment fails and the patient dies.

There exist well-known *affective stances* that accompany ineffectively shared control of disease and treatment (Friedman, 1980). While these psychosocial positions are often part of healthy coping strategies, more commonly they can be defensive maneuvers that aggravate rather than resolve the basic issue of control. Weisman (1976) most thoroughly addresses these "vulnerability variables." He indicates that patients who present with high measures of hopelessness, turmoil, frustration, depression, powerlessness, anxiety, exhaustion, worthlessness, isolation, denial, and repudiation of others tend to have shorter than expected survivals. Conversely, patients who make their needs known and interact with significant others, including staff, tend to live longer than expected (Weisman and Worden, 1975). This focus on active engagement as a means toward survival, increased self-control, and satisfaction is echoed by others (Bahnson, 1975; Derogatis et al., 1976: Gottheil et al., 1979; Nelson et al., 1978; Payne and Krant, 1969; Schmale, 1976).

It is striking and logical that the same patient distress variables are identical for caregivers. As they daily face anxiety, depression, and frustration, they disengage in defense (Adsit, 1977; Koocher, 1979; Vachon et al., 1978). The results are withdrawal, isolation, denial of their own pain and that of patients and colleagues, and displacement of anger and hostility. Most importantly, they perceive themselves as powerless.

When patients lack *power*, they experience an intensification of physical and psychological symptoms (Weisman and Sobel, 1979) stemming from anxiety that nothing will change for them. They respond with anger and make efforts to reduce their distress by gaining power. They demand information and participation in their lives and treatment and demand accountability from caregivers. Patients benefit from information and participation (Brewin, 1977; Krant and Johnston, 1977; Schain, 1980) and are dissatisfied when not supplied it in a reasonable manner (McIntosh, 1974; Schulz and Aderman, 1976). If they are rebuked in their attempts to engage with staff, they may give up and manifest signs of helplessness and hopelessness. In either instance, whether symptoms increase or the patient withdraws because he lacks power, the treatment becomes suboptimal, and effectiveness is diminished.

Staff difficulties with power are similar to those of their patients. When confronted with demands from patients and colleagues in a disturbed system, staff anxiety and anger increase. They then displace anger upward by declaring their colleagues to be inadequate and by demanding that they do better and more, or they displace anger downward by attacking patients for their noncompliance with their treatment and for their painful demands. As others have noted (Baider, 1975; Cassileth and Lief, 1979; Kleiman et al., 1977), caregivers behave according to what the system expects of them. Patients and caregivers mirror each others' maladaptive behaviors and violate their own intentions.

In effect, medical staff create and perpetuate the system that they believe oppresses. They then feel as hopeless and helpless as do their patients.

The current existence of dysfunctional *communication patterns* within the oncology system is, in fact, the social underpinning of struggles with control, affect, and power as givers and receivers of care. All participants experience frustration in attempts to communicate effectively. A major source of frustration is the fragmentation and lack of cohesiveness in the cancer care system. The system's rules demand contradictory behaviors of all participants. Radiotherapy personnel are disapproved when they openly challenge the paradoxes inherent in their practice (Baider, 1975). The advances and subspecialization that permit improved technical care also have negative effects. Research (Baider, 1975; Hayes, 1976; Leopold, 1979; Schulz and Aderman, 1976) shows that patients and families strongly resent the impersonal nature of the system and are directly critical of caregivers.

As professionals, radiation personnel also resent the same system that fosters exclusive, inadequate information dissemination (Greenwald, 1980; Leopold, 1979; McIntosh, 1974; Sheldon et al., 1970; Vachon et al., 1978). They then distort the information they do have (Brewin, 1977; Krant and Johnston, 1977), which in turn affects treatment decisions and their approach toward patients and families. This is fueled by legitimate, competing perspectives concerning the nature and priorities of treatment that push specialties apart. Added to this are ambiguous role definitions that involve real overlap in functions and that have produced no shared awareness of who is accountable to whom, for what, and why. Those directly involved in patient care, who require the most information and support, often receive the least. The responsibility and stress of treatment for any one patient is not possible for a given team member to handle alone and becomes overwhelming when there is faulty communication. Ineffectively shared communication results in breakdown of patients, caregivers, and the system as a whole, and the vicious cycle begins again.

ATTEMPTS AT SOLUTIONS

As the authors have identified issues that emerge in the

literature, as well as in their practice, they similarly identify trends in activities aimed at addressing them. Proposed solutions have arisen out of every discipline in the system and have been directed at remedies not only for a given discipline but for other subgroups as well. The various strategies can best be conceptualized schematically:

CANCER CARE SYSTEM

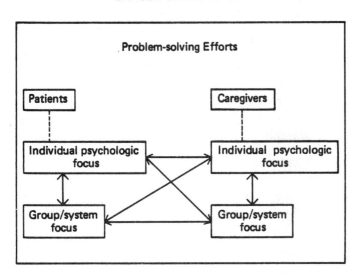

The diagram shows that some efforts exist in a solitary realm, while others overlap and connect with activities in related spheres, crossing individual/group boundaries and patient/caregiver boundaries. It is critical to underscore that each problem has both a psychological dynamic and a social dynamic, and these dynamics are inextricably interrelated. Patients' and caregivers' intrapyschic conflicts and individual role requirements determine their approach to interaction within a treatment setting. Conversely, the structure of the settings in which one operates can reinforce or undermine approaches to working within a given structure.

The Patient: Individual/Psychologic Focus

Patients must make an intrapsychic shift in order to maximize their self-awareness and their engagement with significant others. They are then able to achieve a sense of mastery of available resources. That mastery subsequently permits a greater quantity and quality of life. Patients' perceptions of increasing responsibility for themselves and belief in self-determination go hand in hand with their ability to confront their illness and accept help from others (Nelson et al., 1978). This can occur most easily when patients have the opportunity to externalize conflicts. When proper communication channels are available to patients for seeking information, discussing their feelings, validating the "truth" of their cancer status, and demystifying death, there is notable decrease in symptomatology (Weisman and Sobel, 1979) and decrease in ambivalence about treatment (Leopold, 1979). There is also increased belief in and acceptance of realistic alternatives by patients, families, and caregivers. Patients' satisfaction with the treatment process increases in proportion to their own participation in it, as they feel themselves to exercise control as experts in living. Needless to say, this intrapsychic shift can occur only when patients' needs are met with matching behaviors on the caregivers' part (Gottheil et al., 1979; Koocher, 1979).

The Caregiver: Individual/Psychologic Focus

In caregivers there is an acknowledgment that they must confront their own concerns about death in order to maintain constructive interaction with their patients. The authors derive from the literature and their experience several conclusions. First, physicians, in particular, repeatedly discuss their defenses as obstacles that interfere with their ability to function effectively (Bahnson, 1975; Clark, 1976; Koocher, 1979; Konior and Levine, 1975; Krant and Sheldon, 1971; Schmale, 1976). They indicate a need to live with their vulnerability, tolerate their patients' projections, dependency, and demands, and confront what cancer means to them personally in order to believe in themselves as caregivers. Resolution of these issues allows them to project confidence in themselves to patients, with concurrent sustained involvement, interaction, and satisfaction (Creech, 1975; Greenwald, 1980; Hazra et al., 1977; Schmale, 1976). This permits identification of and intervention with high-risk patients (Bleeker, 1978; Plumb and Holland, 1977; Weisman, 1976) so that treatment is maximally effective. Decision making about individual patients is then based on the experience of the clinician rather than on his uncorrected, idiosyncratic (and often defensive) ideas (Baider, 1975; Greenwald, 1980; Hayes, 1976; McIntosh, 1974; Novack et al., 1979).

After an altered framework of personal/professional goals is adopted, caregivers are free to encourage responsibility on the patients' part. This third area fulfills the patients' request for increased participation (Brown et al., 1976; Cassileth et al., 1980; Weisman, 1976). Patient/caregiver needs are then congruous, and they can give information in a timely and technically skillful way that is in tune with the needs of a particular patient or family. Direct access to staff is highly valued by patients and families; as they humanize themselves as caregivers and assign more control to their patients, the patients feel self-assured and assume increasing responsibility for their part in treatment, abusing staff less (Schmale, 1976). Thus, what initially appears to be irrelevant, threatening, and/or time-consuming actually makes work easier, that is, the redefinition of the nature of medical staff control and reattribution of legitimate control to the patients.

The Patient: Group/System Focus

Adams (1979) suggests that mutual support groups flourish in areas where professional help has been least effective and attainable, i.e. in the case of stigmatizing illnesses. Such groups exhibit modeling and sharing; as patients act as counselors to others like themselves, they help themselves as well. In oncology, this phenomenon ranges from unplanned casual exchanges among patients to formation of well-established self-help groups. Institutionalized caregivers have followed on the heels of their patients, and there is now evidence of a variety of formally and informally structured groups for patients under the auspices of hospitals and private practices. These include patient-family groups (Baker, 1977; Kelly and Asby, 1979), multiple family group therapy (Corder and Anders, 1974; Wellisch et al., 1978), patient-only groups (Kelly and Asby, 1979; Spiegel and Yalom, 1978; Whitman et al., 1979), and patients trained by professionals to counsel patients (Keeling, 1976; Kleiman et al., 1977). These groups operate with various constellations of caregiver leadership, i.e. nurses, psychologists, physicians, social workers, technologists, psychiatrist, chaplains, and even office staff.

Spiegel and Yalom (1978) identify four features inherent in group activity that are not available in individual treatment: universality, altruism, instillation of hope, and group cohesiveness. Beneficial results of the group process are patients' beliefs and activities in their own improvement; lower rates of disease recurrence in patients who have group support (Vachon et al., 1977); another vehicle for externalization of conflicts; a new mechanism for facilitation of patient-caregiver cooperation; an opportunity for reinforcement of a factual and realistic approach to illness; an arena to share concrete resources; an opportunity to acquire new health behavior (Enelow, 1976); insurance against feelings of isolation and uniqueness; and finally, patients' education of professionals about the cancer experience (Keeling, 1976). Caregivers have significantly benefitted from patients' organizing themselves, because as patients share information, losses, and gains with one another, they defuse the pressure upon caregivers to bear all the responsibility for treatment outcome.

The Caregiver: Group/System Focus

Caregivers, by virtue of the multidisciplinary nature of oncology practice, have historically come together in groups through consultation, rounds, and medically oriented conferences. Only recently, however, have they realized that there is still such overwhelming fragmentation of care that supportive groups might help them cope with this inherent stress. Development of a holistic focus in medical education (Cassileth and Egan, 1979; Hayes, 1976), psychosocial training for oncology fellows (Artiss and Levine, 1973; Wise, 1977), multidisciplinary patient care conferences (Bahnson, 1975; Krant and Sheldon, 1971; Parker et al., 1978), psychiatric consultation in oncology (Leopold, 1979), and therapylike groups for staff (Schulz and Aderman, 1976) are phenomena that parallel patients' groups. The benefits are both psychological and social for all involved, and these groups are most effective when there is equal responsibility among members for the participation in the group process outcome.

In a psychological sense, communication that cuts across

boundaries of discipline and hierarchical status has impressive results. An altered perspective of the roles and limitations of any specialty suggests diminished omnipotence but also a decreased sense of despair and responsibility for treatment failures. Awareness that other team members share identical feelings of isolation, helplessness, depression, and frustration can result in avoidance of displacement of anger onto fellow team members (Derogatis et al., 1976; Vachon et al., 1978), and increased knowledge and appreciation of colleagues' actual areas of expertise. Additionally, when group members are open about their shared discomforts, there is a decrease in competition among them, a new ability to redefine their own and others' problems, and an increase in satisfaction and cohesiveness (Braatz and Goudsmit, 1977; Cassileth, 1979; Lansky et al., 1976; Wise, 1977). The result is increasing interaction among caregivers and patients and mutual respect for realistic boundaries (Clark, 1976; Creech, 1975; Krant and Sheldon, 1971; Leopold, 1979).

In a social sense, group support among caregivers has far-ranging effects upon the larger system. As group members feel more confident, they together can give and receive information more accurately and use it more appropriately. They are increasingly open to using other professionals, as well as creatively taking advantage of existing resources (Ryan and Neuenshwander, 1977). Most of all, they recognize their individual limits and coordinate themselves and their treatment more effectively. In essence, mutual support networks among caregivers can provide role clarification and security about their own skills; their accurate perception by colleagues permits comfort when they overlap in their jobs. The effect is that they change the structures that promoted the original denial and suppression of legitimate feelings through their redefined, improved interactions among themselves.

PRINCIPLES OF REORGANIZATION

The patient care team has evolved as the most synthesized practical effort to incorporate the attempted solutions just discussed. Several authors have reported their experiences in developing teams and have identified both rewards and problems

(Bahnson, 1975; Enelow, 1976; Friedman, 1980; Holland, 1976; Koch and Donaldson, 1975; Krant et al., 1976; Lansky et al., 1976; Lehmann et al., 1978; Ryser et al., 1971; Sheldon et al., 1970).

The patient care team can be viewed in terms of its *components, coordination,* and *collaboration.* The *components* of a team are, by definition, its various membership groups. These disciplines need not be an officially constituted body, separately funded, or administratively organized by nonparticipants (Braatz and Goudsmit, 1977). What is essential is that a team mutually and explicitly define itself as a functioning group. Team members must then present themselves in a manner that reflects "consistency, availability, and expertise" commensurate with their specific professions and their status as members of a defined group (McKenzie, 1978). For patients and families, awareness that a treatment team exists, especially if patients are included as participants, results in improved ratings of their own care (Carey and Posavac, 1979; Krant and Johnston, 1977; McIntosh, 1974).

The concept of a team implies existence of a procedure whereby individual efforts are coordinated in some fashion. This minimally involves periodic joint meetings of all team members to review information and treatment planning. Coordination insures the best chance to meet patients' needs by (1) allowing opportunities to discuss material presented by patients to various staff in multiple ways (Krant and Sheldon, 1971; Lansky et al., 1976), (2) detecting inconsistencies and distortions in staff perception of patients (McKenzie, 1978; Payne and Krant, 1969), (3) preventing dislocation, depersonalization, abandonment, and avoidance of patients when treatment interventions change (Creech, 1975; Dunphy, 1976), (4) facilitating reinforcement and repetition of information given to patients by staff, (5) reducing the quality and quantity of stress placed upon any team member by a particular patient, and (6) allowing patients and families a legitimate channel through which to address questions and concerns about any facet of their care, thereby minimizing defensiveness and/or disengagement on their parts.

Even when a team is well coordinated, its value for staff is shaped by the *nature of their collaboration.* Schain's discussion concerning "shared responsibility" between patient and physician is equally applicable to exchanges among team members; movement is geared toward "a mutual endeavor between two parties who are dedicated to the effective management of a problem . . . based on mutual respect and collaborative communication" (Schain, 1980). This model assumes that each party has a unique and an essential body of information, with a responsibility to exchange that information in a "cross-party" process that demands initiation and reception of communication by all parties. This type of interaction has otherwise been referred to as "unstratified collaboration" (Cassileth, 1979) and "egalitarian rather than traditionally hierarchical" (Ryser et al., 1971), in which a "democratic sharing of responsibilities can take place" (Bahnson, 1975). Parkes (1974) best captures the process in his assertion that "What is needed is a mutually supportive therapeutic community in which the emotional needs of patients, relatives and staff are recognized and met. In such a setting, communication about the illness is seen as an important matter, responsibility for which is shared by the staff team" (p. 190).

In fact, when team members approach one another on equal footing, interchanges are possible that cannot exist in an authoritarian structure. The advantages of democratic teamwork, affectively and technically, can be summarized as follows. *Affectively,* periodic opportunities to consensually validate concerns help to "intensify a sense of colleagueship, itself comforting and productive of maximum team effort (Leopold, 1979, p. 261). In authoritarian settings, anger and frustration of team members are rarely overtly expressed but rather take the form of detached professionalism and abandonment of the patient (Clark, 1976), ultimately eroding the self-confidence of caregivers when they chronically internalize such feelings. The team is a mechanism that can facilitate open handling of commonly experienced intrapersonal conflicts and interpersonal differences. When dissonance is directly handled, decreased covert expression of frustration, increased insight into one's own limitations, and a sense of mutual support result. Belonging to a supportive team that shares mutual rewards prevents the team from withdrawing from patients, from each other, and from the tasks at hand. In a *technical* sense, when all disciplines, including the patients, are recognized as crucial in the organization and planning of treatment, joint decision making can occur throughout treatment. Obviously, this means that discontinuities in care can be avoided and that specific interventions can be well thought out rather than be applied in emergency stopgap fashion. Greenwald (1980) shows that physicians and nurses often fail to agree on their respective responsibilities for providing emotional support for the patient, with the consequence that their perceptions of what they are providing are faulty or inaccurate. The implication is that exploring with patients their views of their illness is a responsibility of all team members (Krant and Sheldon, 1971; Lansky et al., 1976). Koch and Donaldson (1975) point out that "paradoxically, this structural interdisciplinary collaboration does not lead to role diffusion, but to role clarity, and enhanced awareness of one's particular expertise" (p. 318).

Thus, we see that such a team has implicit in it the structural components and theoretical intimations that allow radiotherapy staff to derive a new set of principles around which to reorganize their practice. The authors share the view that "basic changes in the authority system surrounding cancer treatment will have to take place before other caretakers can perform an expanded support role reliably and effectively" (Greenwald, 1980, p. 185). The predominant mode of patient/caregiver activity has fostered patients' being accountable to staff without staff being answerable to them. This takes place in an organization in which caregivers ask accountability of one another without being equally accountable in turn. In essence, medical personnel are authoritarian not only with their patients but with one another as well. We have seen the results of activities governed by such principles: Patients become inappropriately submissive, noncompliant, and/or demanding. They play themselves against any or all of staff, staff against them, and staff against each other. As Cassileth (1979) describes, in dysfunctional treatment units, "Individual hostility is displaced in a fashion that mirrored and intensified existing hierarchical relationships." Intensification of conflicts through upward or downward displacement results in a situation in which no party can conceive of resolution. Individuals deny their existence as creators and perpetuators of "the system."

When patients and caregivers take the position that they are responsible for neither their illnesses nor the disturbance of the treatment system, they vacillate between two defensive postures: They place excessive blame outside of themselves — anger — or they place excessive blame within themselves — depression. Any realistic chance for change becomes theoretically and practically impossible due to individuals' basic confusion about themselves and the treatment process.

In a psychological sense, "good copers" (Weisman, 1976; Weisman and Sobel, 1979; Weisman and Worden, 1976) function in what the authors would term a democratic fashion. They confront issues openly and directly, redefine their problems in the context of their situation, cooperate actively rather than passively, and insist on more information when needed for better treatment. "Bad copers" function in what the authors would term an authoritarian fashion. They defensively seek to maintain an unchanged status by trying to obliterate their disturbed feelings without accurate recognition of or resolution of the inciting problem. Needless to say, there are democratic and authoritarian caregivers as well.

Democratic patients and caregivers *organize around the following principles* concerning themselves and the treatment process:

1. *Both patients and caregivers are equally responsible for the outcome of treatment.* The nature of an individual's responsibility is determined by the special skills and needs he has as a participant in the treatment team. This implies that everyone is as responsible to himself, to insure his own well-being, as he is to his patients and colleagues to insure theirs. When he assumes more than his share of responsibility, he overburdens himself and deprives others of potential gains and losses. When he assumes less than his share of responsibility, he overburdens others and robs himself of potential gains and losses.

2. *Both patients and caregivers are accountable to each other during the treatment process, in accord with the responsibilities they actually carry.* Insofar as power or control is shared, so, too, open answerability to each other must take place. Otherwise, one invites dysfunctional accounting

on the parts of patients and colleagues, that is, they either defer excessively or become angry. In either case, the communication necessary for effective treatment breaks down.

3. *Optimal treatment outcome, affective well-being, and satisfaction occur when the maximum possible input in decision making is secured from all team members at any point in the treatment process.* This assumes that all team members, even when they appear impaired in their functioning, can contribute something substantial and meaningful to the treatment process. Team distress and dysfunction can best be prevented by shared assumption of responsibility for problems inherent in the treatment process. In the same measure, the rewards of treatment can be mutually distributed and enjoyed.

The authors believe that adoption of this perspective of shared control, power, responsibility, and accountability is desirable and the only realistic way to make the current system work for its members. It is only within the context of a democratic, well-functioning group that individuals can achieve a heightened awareness of themselves and their roles.

IMPLICATIONS FOR RADIATION ONCOLOGY PRACTICE

Specific radiation oncology literature and the experiences of radiotherapy staff exemplify issues and solutions in oncology practice at large. Patients have little reliable information about radiation therapy when they come for treatment. They find their referring physicians deficient in providing even basic information about the frequency and procedure of treatment, as well as its efficacy (Lehman et al., 1978; Peck and Boland, 1977). Many patients believe that treatment is inherently damaging, carcinogenic, and/or noncurative (Peck and Boland, 1977). Patients experience high levels of anxiety and depression at the onset of treatment (Adsit, 1977; Fobair, 1977; Holland et al., 1979; Mitchell and Glicksman, 1977; Peck and Boland, 1977; Rotman et al., 1977; Smith and McNamara, 1977). This tends to drop off rapidly and remain manageable during treatment. The reasons for this are (1) corrective information shared with patients about their disease and the treatment process, (2) frequent patient access to multiple caregivers, (3) patients' exposure to other patients with whom to share their experience, (4) readily available medical attention when problems arise, and (5) patients' belief that they are actively doing something to control their diseases. To be added is that patients experience a sense of well-being associated with "the relative compositional stability of the team" (Mitchell and Glicksman, 1977).

The authors find that their patients' anxiety and depression often escalate at the end of their treatment course, and they agree with Holland et al. (1979) that this resurgence of dysphoric affect stems from patients' anticipation of loss of relationships with staff, loss of close monitoring, and perception of increased vulnerability to their disease. These feelings are dramatically intensified when (1) continuity of care is not assured with the radiation oncology team, (2) there is inadequate preparation for patients' smooth transition to other oncology caregivers (Brewin, 1977; Krant and Sheldon, 1971), and (3) when patients end a course of radiotherapy without a sound and realistic understanding of its value in the context of their overall treatment. The authors have seen almost complete loss of cognitive and affective gains in patients during therapy when they do not promote carry-over and follow-up.

Some patients ask too few questions of radiotherapy staff, and others demand excessive attention from any and all. Both behaviors point to two inadequacies in practice: First, as individual caregivers, radiotherapy personnel have not matched their intervention to the coping style of their patients and families; second, as a team, they have not coordinated and reinforced each other's efforts. That patients experience dissonance is a reflection of individual and interteam conflicts; however, few patients are dissatisfied with their treatment or unusually anxious or depressed when staff attend to these needs.

As caregivers, radiotherapy staff can only attend to patients' needs when they meet minimum criteria for practice. These criteria assume that staff are psychologically comfortable in working with cancer patients and that they have confidence in their abilities to work with other team members. In radiation oncology practice, they are responsible, at the very least, for—

1. skilled and responsible execution of the technical aspects of their jobs;
2. willingness to embrace the inherent overlap in the non-technical aspects of their jobs.

If they practice with great individual technical expertise but do not acknowledge and validate the work of fellow team members, the team will function in an exclusionary and hierarchical fashion. When they combine technical expertise with an expanded appreciation of and utilization of other team members' contributions, their practice will be inclusionary and democratic. The democratic process automatically incorporates patients' and staff's psychosocial needs.

Table 14-I suggests some typical traditional functions of team members and possible expanded redefinition of their roles.

When one practices in a traditional technical fashion, treatment is likely to be fragmented and impersonal. The physician is more likely to assume too much control and responsibility (Ryser et al., 1971), some of which should be shared with other team members. Radiotherapy personnel are more likely to treat the disease rather than the patient. When the definition of practice is expanded, several themes emerge. Staff members interact with each other more frequently in psychosocial as well as technical aspects of patient care (Brown et al., 1976; Lansky et al., 1976). This encourages initiation of communication by all team members. Staff draws upon the wealth of information about their patients and their practice that they assimilate in the process of performing technical tasks. They notice that they overlap in functions as providers of support to patients, families, and each other. In sum, when radiotherapy personnel perceive themselves beyond traditional definitions of task-oriented roles, they respect each others' expertise, collaborate in a collegial, rather than deferential or authoritarian, fashion, and share the positives and negatives of their efforts.

The only barriers to such reorganization in radiation oncology are a distorted sense of identity as individual professionals and maintenance of a defensive posture regarding overlapping role definition. Once these barriers are overcome, a shift in clinical practice is readily achieved. The basic components of a team

Table 14-I
RADIATION ONCOLOGY TEAM

	Traditional/Technical Roles	*Expanded Roles*
Technologist	1. set up fields according to physicians' calculations 2. deliver the dose to the patient 3. operate equipment safely	1. due to understanding of disease process and treatment effects, identify and refer medical concerns to team members 2. due to close contact between technologist and patients/families, identify patients'/families' psychosocial needs and support and/or refer to team members
Nurse	1. assist with physical exam and care along with physician 2. coordinate laboratory and diagnostic procedures 3. identify evolving medical problems 4. aid in stomal and nutritional support	1. support and educate other team members, hospital staff, and community 2. educate and counsel patients and families 3. screen patients'/families' concerns and support and/or refer to team members
Social Worker	1. screen patients and families for eligibility for concrete services 2. provide support services and refer to outside agencies or team members when necessary 3. assist patients and families in overall coordination of care	1. gather information from team members about aspects of patients' care 2. reinforce activities of the rest of the team with patients and families 3. collaborate with team and hospital staff to coordinate patients' care 4. support and educate other team members in psychosocial interactions
Radiation Oncologist	1. direct and determine treatment as team leader 2. make all major treatment and management decisions 3. identify and manage treatment complications	1. gather information from team members about aspects of patients' care 2. reinforce activities of the rest of the team with patients and families 3. actively collaborate with team and outside oncology caregivers in comprehensive cancer care planning and continuing care 4. represent radiation oncology team to cancer care system and to community

already exist, and it is easy to coordinate efforts because the members are geographically self-contained and their numbers are sufficiently small to permit frequent and inclusive joint interchanges.

A more difficult task of a radiation oncology team within the cancer care system is that the goal of democratic practice is challenged by organizational and psychological obstacles. In a purely logistical sense, the sheer number and variety of caregivers are so great that organization of care becomes "a social engineering project" (Walter, 1979). Gathering and coordinating data are difficult but possible with concerted effort.

The more fundamental issues that prevent shared power and control in the system are the distorted perceptions caregivers have of themselves and their colleagues. Historically, radiation therapy and surgery were the original and major modes of cancer treatment. In recent years, with advances in the use of cytotoxic agents, medical oncology has grown exponentially and has come to the foreground of modern cancer therapy. An unintended by-product of this development is that the *consultative* nature of radiation oncology has been underscored by both surgeons and medical oncologists. They frequently focus on the technical aspects of radiotherapeutic expertise and treat the professionals involved as adjuvant or palliative agents of treatment. As is common with individuals who have felt oppressed but have then risen to the level of their oppressors, medical oncologists and surgeons seem to resent radiation oncologists for having had primacy in cancer treatment in the past; they strive to move beyond them and establish primacy for themselves. The natural response is for radiotherapists to try to shift the locus of control of treatment back to themselves. This process is competitive and conflictual for all caregivers and nonproductive of optimal patient care. It bears striking resemblance to the dysfunctional behaviors among patients and caregivers and among patient care team members.

This is compounded by radiation oncologists' contradictory perceptions of themselves. They want the luxury to function as consultants, who provide a time-limited, highly specialized technical service, but they wish to provide varying forms of clinical care for the patients undergoing treatment and to be respected as rightful participants in the process of continuing management and planning. In reality, they have the skills and the responsibility to do both. What often occurs, however, is that they resist providing clinical care for their patients when they become less definitive and more palliative, and suffer physical and psychological distress. They prefer medical oncologists to take over when patients become too compromised. It is not difficult to understand why colleagues tend to escalate efforts to assume primacy over treatment and relegate secondary importance to radiotherapists as technicians. The point is that radiotherapists must accurately perceive and consistently demonstrate both technical expertise *and* knowledge and willingness to participate in clinical care. By the same token, medical oncologists and surgeons must recognize the nature and limits of their technical skills and of their particular responsibilities for primary patient care. Failure to correct distortions of themselves and of one another will perpetuate the existing defensiveness, hostility, and exclusionary politics of treatment. What is required is a mutually corrected definition of each other. It is only then that all can equitably share power, control, responsibility, and accountability. This will improve the treatment of patients and realize the goal of productive engagement with one another as a cancer care team.

It is possible to experience a new respect for each other's opinions, to encourage collaboration around areas of expertise, and to actualize the optimal cancer care that arises from the joint practice of all disciplines. The result will be to engage the teams in planned, cooperative, and continuing patient care. Both personally and professionally, as individuals and groups, the products of this democratic process are healthier and happier patients and more effective, efficient, and satisfied caregivers.

REFERENCES

Adams, J. 1979. Mutual-help Groups: Enhancing the Coping Ability of Oncology Clients. *Cancer Nursing, 2(2)*:95-98.

Adsit, C.G., Jr. 1977. The Radiation Therapist. *Archives of the Foundation of Thanatology, 6(2)*.

Artiss, K.L. and A.S. Levine. 1973. Doctor-Patient Relation in Severe Illness: A Seminar for Oncology Fellows. *New England Journal of Medicine, 288 (23)*:1210-1214.

Bahnson, C.B. 1975. Psychologic and Emotional Issues in Cancer: The Psychotherapeutic Care of the Cancer Patient. *Seminars in Oncology, 2(4)*:293-309.

Baider, L. 1975. Private Experience and Public Expectation on the Cancer Ward. *Omega: Journal of Death and Dying, 6(4)*:373-81.

Baker, K. 1977. Oncology Support Groups for Out-patients. *Hospital Topics,* *55(1):*40-42.

Belknap, R. 1977. A Dying Patient. *Synthesis, 1(1):*156-60.

Bleeker, J.A.C. 1978-79. Brief Psychotherapy with Lung Patients. *Psychotherapy and Psychosomatics, 29(1-4):*282-87.

Braatz, G.A. and A. Goudsmit. 1977. A Multidisciplinary Approach to Cancer Care. *Archives of the Foundation of Thanatology, 6(2).*

Brewin, T.B. 1977. The Cancer Patient: Communication and Morale. *British Medical Journal, 2:*1623-27.

Brown, N.K., M.A. Brown, and D. Thompson. 1976. Decision-making for the Terminally Ill Patient. In J.W. Cullen et al., *Cancer: The Behavioral Dimensions.* New York: Raven, pp. 319-329.

Carey, R.G. and E. J. Posavac. 1979. Holistic Care in a Cancer Care Center. *Nursing Research, 28(4):*213-226.

Cassileth, B.R. 1979. Specialization and Holistic Care. In B.R. Cassileth, *The Cancer Patient: Social and Medical Aspects of Care.* Philadelphia: Lea and Febiger, pp. 283-300.

Cassileth, B.R. and T.A. Egan. 1979. Modification of Medical Student Perceptions of the Cancer Experience. *Journal of Medical Education, 54(10):* 797-802.

Cassileth, B.R. and H.L. Lief. 1979. Cancer: A Biopsychosocial Model. In B.R. Cassileth, *The Cancer Patient: Social and Medical Aspects of Care.* Philadelphia: Lea and Febiger, pp. 17-31.

Cassileth, B.R., R.V. Zupkis, K. Sutton-Smith, and V. March. 1980. Information and Participation Preferences Among Cancer Patients. *Annals of Internal Medicine, 92(6):*832-36.

Clark, R.L. 1976. Psychologic Reactions of Patients and Health Professionals to Cancer. In J.W. Cullen et al., *Cancer: The Behavioral Dimensions.* New York: Raven, pp. 1-10.

Corder, M.P. and R.L. Anders. 1974. Death and Dying—Oncology Discussion Group. *Journal of Psychiatric Nursing, 12(4):*10-14.

Craig, T.J., and M.D. Abeloff. 1974. Psychiatric Symptomatology Among Hospitalized Cancer Patients. *American Journal of Psychiatry, 13(12):*1323-27.

Creech, R.H. 1975. The Psychologic Support of the Cancer Patient: A Medical Oncologist's Viewpoint. *Seminars in Oncology, 2(4):*285-92.

Dansak, D.A. and R.S. Cordas. 1978-79. Cancer: Denial or Suppression. *International Journal of Psychiatry-Medicine, 9(3-4):*257-62.

Derogatis, L.R., M.D. Abeloff, and C.D. McBeth. 1976. Cancer Patients and Their Physicians in the Perception of Psychological Symptoms. *Psychosomatics, 17(4):*197-201.

Derogatis, L.R., M.D. Abeloff, N. Melisaratos. 1979. Psychological Coping Mechanisms and Survival Time in Metastatic Breast Cancer. *Journal of the American Medical Association, 242(14):*1504-1508.

Dunphy, J.E. 1976. Annual Discourse on Caring for the Patient with Cancer.

*New England Journal of Medicine, 295(6):*313-19.

Enelow, A.J. 1976. Group Influences on Health Behavior: A Social Learning Perspective. In J.W. Cullen et al., *Cancer: The Behavioral Dimensions.* New York: Raven, pp. 63-83.

Fobair, P. 1977. Group Work with Cancer Patients in Radiation Therapy. *Archives of the Foundation of the Foundation of Thanatology, 6(2).*

Forester, B.M., D.S. Kornfeld, and J. Fleiss. 1978. Psychiatric Aspects of Radiotherapy. *American Journal of Psychiatry, 135(8):*960-63.

Franzino, M., J.J. Geren, and G.L. Meiman. 1976. Group Discussion Among the Terminally Ill. *International Journal of Group Psychotherapy, 26(1):*43-48.

Friedman, B.D. 1980. Coping with Cancer: A Guide for Health Care Professionals. *Cancer Nursing, 3(2):*105-110.

Glicksman, A.S., G. Mitchell, and C. Geyer. 1977. Psychosocial Implications of Radiotherapy. *Archives of the Foundation of Thanatology, 6(2).*

Gottheil, E., C. McGurn-Wealtha, and O. Pollak. 1979. Awareness and Disengagement in Cancer Patients. *American Journal of Psychiatry, 136(5):* 632-36.

Greenwald, H.P. 1980. *Social Problems in Cancer Control.* Cambridge, Massachusetts: Ballinger.

Hayes, D.M. 1976. The Impact of the Health Care Systems on Physician Attitudes and Behaviors. In J.W. Cullen et al., *Cancer: The Behavioral Dimensions.* New York: Raven, pp. 145-69.

Hazra, T.A., C. Rose, and V. Rose. 1977. Psychological Problems of Patients Receiving Radiotherapy. *Archives of the Foundation of Thanatology, 6(2).*

Holland, J.C. 1976. Coping with Cancer: A Challenge to the Behavioral Sciences. In J.W. Cullen et al., *Cancer: The Behavioral Dimensions.* New York: Raven, pp. 263-68.

Holland, J.C. 1977. Psychological Aspects of Oncology. *Medical Clinics of North America, 61(4):*737-48.

Holland, J.C., J. Rowland, A. Lebovits, and R. Rusalem. 1979. Reactions to Cancer Treatment: Assessment of Emotional Response to Adjuvant Radiotherapy as a Guide to Planned Intervention. *Psychiatric Clinics of North America, 2(2):*347-58.

Keeling, W. 1976. Live the Pain, Learn the Hope: A Beginner's Guide to Cancer Counseling. *Personnel and Guidance Journal, 54(10):*502-506.

Kelly, P.P. and G.C. Asby. 1979. Group Approaches for Cancer Patients: Establishing a Group. *American Journal of Nursing, 79(5):*914-915.

Kleiman, M.A., J.E. Mantell, and E.S. Alexander. 1977. Rx for Social Death: The Cancer Patient as Counselor. *Community Mental Health Journal, 13(2):*115-24.

Koch, C.R. and M.H. Donaldson. 1975. Psychosocial Care in Malignant Disease of Childhood: Organization and Structural Implications. *Seminars in Oncology, 2(4):*317-21.

Konior, G.S. and A.S. Levine. 1975. The Fear of Dying: How Patients and

Their Doctors Behave. *Seminars in Oncology, 2(4):*311-16.

Koocher, G.P. 1979. Adjustment and Coping Strategies Among the Caretakers of Cancer Patients. *Social Work in Health Care, 5(2):*145-50.

Krant, M.J. 1976. Problems of the Physician in Presenting the Patient with the Diagnosis. In J.W. Cullen et al., *Cancer: The Behavioral Dimensions.* New York: Raven, pp. 269-74.

Krant, M.J., M. Beiser, and G. Adler. 1976. The Role of a Hospital-based Psychosocial Unit in Terminal Cancer, Illness, and Bereavement. *Journal of Chronic Diseases, 29(2):*115-27.

Krant, M.J. and L. Johnston. 1977-78. Family Members' Perceptions of Communications in Late Stage Cancer. *International Journal of Psychiatry in Medicine, 8(2):*203-16.

Krant, M.J. and A. Sheldon. 1971. The Dying Patient—Medicine's Responsibility. *Journal of Thanatology, 1(1):*1-24.

Lansky, S.B., J.T. Lowman, J. Gyulay, and K. Briscoe. 1976. A Team Approach to Coping with Cancer. In J.W. Cullen et al., *Cancer: The Behavioral Dimensions.* New York: Raven, pp. 291-317.

Lehmann, J.F., M.A. Delisa, C.G. Warren, B.J. Delateur, P.L. Bryant, and C.G. Nicholson. 1978. Cancer Rehabilitation: Assessment of Need, Development and Evaluation of a Model of Care. *Archives of Physical Medicine and Rehabilitation, 59(9):*410-19.

Leopold, R.L. 1979. The Role of the Psychiatrist. In B.R. Cassileth, *The Cancer Patient: Social and Medical Aspects of Care.* Philadelphia: Lea and Febiger, pp. 249-65.

Lichtenberg, P. On Responsibility. In *Toward Equality: Up and Against.* Unpublished essays. Canaday Library, Bryn Mawr College, Bryn Mawr, Pennsylvania.

McIntosh, J. 1974. Processes of Communication, Information Seeking, and Control Associated with Cancer: A Selective Review of the Literature. *Social Science and Medicine, 8(4):*167-87.

McKenzie, S. 1978. The Cancer Care Team in the Community Hospital. *Supervisor Nurse, 9(8):*20-22.

Mitchell, G.W. and A.S. Glicksman. 1977. Cancer Patients: Knowledge and Attitudes. *Cancer, 40(1):*61-66.

Nelson, W.A., L.H. Maurer, and P.Q. Harris. 1978. Living Before Death with Chronic Cancer. *Archives of the Foundation of Thanatology, 7(2).*

Novack, D.H., R. Plumer, R.L. Smith, I.T. Ochitell, G.R. Morrow, and J.M. Bennett. 1979. Changes in Physicians' Attitudes Toward Telling the Cancer Patient. *Journal of the American Medical Association, 241(9):*897-900.

Parker, E., S. Bailis, L. Nathanson, and M. Costanza. 1978. The Use of a Multidisciplinary Staff Conference on an Inpatient Medical Oncology Ward. *Archives of the Foundation of Thanatology, 7(2).*

Parkes, C.M. 1974. Comment: Communication and Cancer—A Social Psychiatrist's View. *Social Science and Medicine, 8(4):*189-90.

Parsell, S. and E.M. Tagliareni. 1974. Cancer Patients Help Each Other.

*American Journal of Nursing, 74(4):*650-51.

Payne, E.C., Jr., and M. Krant. 1969. The Psychosocial Aspects of Advanced Cancer: Teaching Simple Interviewing Techniques and Record Keeping. *Journal of American Medical Association, 210(7):*1238-42.

Peck, A. and J. Boland. 1977. Emotional Reactions to Radiation Treatment. *Cancer, 40(1):*180-84.

Perez, C.A., L.A. Hanns, N. Sedrunsk, and L. Braun. 1977. Psychological Aspects of Cancer and Radiation Therapy. *Archives of the Foundation of Thanatology, 6(2).*

Pilsecker, C. 1979. Terminal Cancer: A Challenge for Social Work. *Social Work in Health Care, 4(4):*369-79.

Plumb, M.M. and J. Holland. 1977. Comparative Studies of Psychological Function in Patients with Advanced Cancer. I: Self-reported Depressive Symptoms. *Psychosomatic Medicine, 39(4):*264-76.

Prior, J. 1976: Communication and the Cancer Patient. *Lancet, 7983:*470.

Rotman, M., L. Rogow, G. DeLeon, and N. Heskel. 1977. Supportive Therapy in Radiation Oncology. *Cancer, 39:*744-50.

Ryan, M.E. and B. Neuenshwander. 1977. Team Approach to Psychological Management of Patients with Neoplastic Disease. *Radiologic Technology, 49(3):*285-89.

Ryser, C.P., A. Sheldon, and C.G. Schwartz. 1971. Problems with Change: The Vicissitudes of a Pilot Comprehensive Cancer Care Program. *Journal of the Foundation of Thanatology, 1(3).*

Sadowski, C.J., S.F. Davis, and M.C. Loftus-Vergari. 1978. Locus of Control and Death Anxiety: A Reexamination. *Omega, 10(3):*203-10.

Schain, W.L. 1980. Patients' Rights in Decision Making: The Case for Personalism vs Paternalism in Health Care. *Cancer, 46:*1035-41.

Schmale, A.H. 1976. Psychological Reactions to Recurrences, Metastases or Disseminated Cancer. *International Journal of Radiation Oncology, Biology, Physics, 1 (5-6):*515-20.

Schnaper, N. 1977. Psychosocial Aspects of Management of the Patient with Cancer. *Medical Clinics of North America, 61(5):*1147-1155.

Schulz, R. and D. Aderman. 1976. How the Medical Staff Copes with Dying Patients: A Critical Review. *Omega, 7(1):*11-21.

Sheldon, A., C.P. Ryser, and M.J. Krant. 1970. An Integrated Family Oriented Cancer Care Program: The Report of a Pilot Project in the Socioemotional Management of Chronic Disease. *Journal of Chronic Diseases, 22(11):*743-55.

Smith, L.L. and J.J. McNamara. 1977. Social Work Services for Radiation Therapy Patients and Their Families. *Hospital and Community Psychiatry, 28(10):*752-54.

Spiegel, D. and I.D. Yalom. 1978. A Support Group for Dying Patients. *International Journal of Group Psychotherapy, 28(2):*233-45.

Vachon, M.L.S., A. Formo, J. Cochrane, W.A.L. Lyall, and J. Rogers. 1977. The Effect of Psychosocial Milieu on Adaptation to Breast Cancer. *Archives of the Foundation of Thanatology, 6(2).*

Vachon, M.L.S., W.A.L. Lyall, and S.J.J. Freeman. 1978. Measurement and Management of Stress in Health Professionals Working with Advanced Cancer Patients. *Death Education, 1(4):*365-75.

Vettesee, J.M. 1976. Problems of the Patient Confronting the Diagnosis of Cancer. In J.W. Cullen et al., *Cancer: The Behavioral Dimensions.* New York: Raven.

Walter, N.T. 1979. Continuing Care of the Cancer Patient as a Social Engineering Problem. *Cancer Research, 39:*2859-62.

Weisman, A.D. 1976. Early Diagnosis of Vulnerability in Cancer Patients. *American Journal of Medicine and Science, 271(2):*187-96.

Weisman, A.D. and H.J. Sobel. 1979. Coping with Cancer Through Self-Instruction: A Hypothesis. *Journal of Human Stress, 5(1):*3-8.

Weisman, A.D. and J.W. Worden. 1975. Psychological Analysis of Cancer Deaths. *Omega, 6(1):*61-75.

Weisman, A.D. and J.W. Worden. 1976-77. The Existential Plight in Cancer: Significance of the First 100 Days. *International Journal of Psychiatry and Medicine, 7(1):*1-15.

Wellisch, D.K., M.B. Mosher, and C. Van Scoy. 1978. Management of Family Emotion Stress: Family Group Therapy in a Private Oncology Practice. *International Journal of Group Psychotherapy, 28(2):*225-31.

Whitman, H.H., J.P. Gustafson, and F.W. Coleman. 1979. Group Approaches for Cancer Patients: Leaders and Members. *American Journal of Nursing, 79(5):*910-13.

Wise, T.N. 1977. Training Oncology Fellows in Psychological Aspects of Their Specialty. *Cancer, 39(6):*2584-87.

_____ Chapter 15 _____

PSYCHOSOCIAL ASPECTS OF RADIATION ONCOLOGY
Training of Residents

KENNETH H. LUK, JOHN W. HARRIS,
NORMAN L. MAGES, AND JOSEPH R. CASTRO

INTRODUCTION

The psychosocial aspects of cancer, and the unique needs of the cancer patients, have attracted increasing interest in recent years. It is recognized that a physician does not deal with cancer as a pathological process only. It is not adequate to deliver good patient care to someone with cancer without considering the psychological and social welfare of that patient. Certainly, high quality medical care requires a well-informed physician making a correct diagnosis through up-to-date tests, giving efficacious treatment by choosing the appropriate therapy programs, and ascertaining the continued welfare of the patient by careful follow-up examinations. However, as Rosenbaum so aptly stated, "... Cancer is not a single disease, and how well a patient lives will be determined by the kind of cancer he has as well as his particular psychological makeup and his body's response to treatment" (Rosenbaum, 1975). In expanding on this concept of the team approach to the care of the cancer patient, he draws on the

_____

Supported in part by the National Institute of Health and the National Cancer Institute, CA 5R18, CA 16873.

123

supportive services of nurses, social services, volunteers, and the clergy, as well as developing programs for exercise and nutrition counseling (Rosenbaum et al., 1978a, 1978b).

Regardless of the adaptational ability of a patient, cancer *is always a catastrophic* illness. The patient's point of view has been eloquently expressed by Fiore in his article that appeared in the *New England Journal of Medicine* in February, 1979. In this article, he recounted his experience with having embryonal cell carcinoma of the testis, his treatments with chemotherapy, and his relationships with his physicians. He gave valuable insights as well as recommendations to physicians who assume the responsibility of cancer patients' care.

Even though more than half of all cancer patients in the United States receive radiation treatments in the course of their illness, either for palliation or for cure, relatively little has been written about the concepts of social needs as they apply to radiation oncology. Peck and Boland (1977) interviewed fifty patients seen at the Radiotherapy Service of the Mount Sinai Medical Center of New York City and reported on the attitudes toward radiotherapy and the way these attitudes were affected by the actual experience of the radiation treatments. The patients had tremendous fears and misconceptions about treatments by radiation as inherently damaging to the patient, and few believed that the treatments could be curative. Rotman et al. (1977) of New York Medical College acknowledged the "misunderstanding, confusion and apprehension" in the use of irradiation in cancer treatments. Based on their experience, they recommended "emotional support prior to and during the course of therapy facilitated by a written interview that allows the radiation oncologist to be a supportive communicator of realistic information."

Among the scant literature regarding the psychosocial aspect of radiation oncology, the authors did not find any mention of an important member of the cancer health care team in the department of radiation oncology, i.e. the radiation oncology resident. This chapter will discuss the role of the resident in caring for the psychosocial needs of cancer patients and suggest specific measures that might be implemented in training programs to prepare better future radiation oncologists.

DEVELOPMENT OF RADIATION ONCOLOGY
RESIDENCY PROGRAMS

Radiation oncology is a newly emerging medical specialty with its roots in general radiology. It began when some radiologists used x-rays and radioactive isotopes in the treatment of malignant tumors, usually as a minor part of their overall practice. With the passage of time, a few of these general radiologists became full-time therapeutic radiologists, and a distinctly new clinical specialty emerged. At that time radiotherapists were more often viewed as button-pushers than as full partners in the surgeon-dominated management team. Dying patients were carted to the dark corners of the basement for radiation treatments to palliate advanced symptoms. Potentially curable patients all received surgery. There is little wonder that radiation therapy still carries the image of hopelessness. With dedicated and scientifically conducted clinical research, however, radiation therapy has demonstrated its usefulness in cancer treatments and has established its position as one of the major cancer treatment modalities.

The specialty of therapeutic radiology eventually weaned itself from general radiology and, in 1934, established a separate specialty board. This process of differentiation has continued, and today radiation oncologists participate broadly in all aspects of cancer care including consultative mangement, follow-up care, education, and research. The increasing preference for the term *radiation oncologist* instead of *radiation therapist* reflects this broader role (Fuller, 1980).

These historical developments have been accompanied by significant changes in radiation oncology residency programs. Initially, major emphasis was placed on the physical and technical aspects of radiation treatments. These skills, including operation of complex machines, techniques of interstitial or intracavitary brachytherapy, calculation of radiation dosage, and delivery of radiation via complicated treatment planning (with the use of computers), remain a major part of residency training today. In addition, the study of the natural history of cancer and the responses of tumors to various modes of treatment is also an essential part of the training of radiation oncologists, even more so as multimodality treatment has become increasingly common. This is particularly important in view of a remarkable growth in the number of medical oncologists being trained and subsequently practicing cancer medicine. The radiation oncology resident has to be trained to relate to this new counterpart, as well as the traditional partners in surgery and family practice. The resident must also acquire a solid foundation in radiobiology and physics, the sciences that underpin his clinical practice and form the basis for research in further advancement of this field.

Given all of this, it is not surprising that very little emphasis has been placed on familiarizing the resident with the psychosocial aspects of radiation oncology. Patients with obvious emotional or psychological needs are usually delegated to the care of social workers. The more severely affected patients with abnormal behaviors can be recognized readily, and these may be referred to psychiatrists. Patients with less obvious needs may not be dealt with at all, since the referring physician may not see the patient during radiation treatments, and the radiation oncologist is often not equipped to deal with such matters.

Although it is demonstrably true that many, if not most, senior faculty members of radiation oncology departments received their own training in an environment that did not stress the psycho-social aspects of patient care, it seems obvious that this deficit in training will be perpetuated unless the need is recognized and steps are taken to correct it.

Table 15-I illustrates a curriculum generally used for radiation oncology residency training in most established institutions. Depending on the strength of the faculties of the institution, emphasis may be placed more on one aspect of the training program than another. To ensure adequate clinical radiotherapy training for the residents, the department of radiation oncology must treat a minimum number of patients per year, with various types of cancers, so that over a three- to four-year period, the resident will be exposed to different situations of clinical diagnosis and treatment. The department must also maintain a follow-up clinic so that the residents will be able to learn from the outcome of radiotherapy whether there have been successes in cure or

Table 15-I

CURRICULUM GENERALLY USED IN RESIDENCY TRAINING PROGRAMS

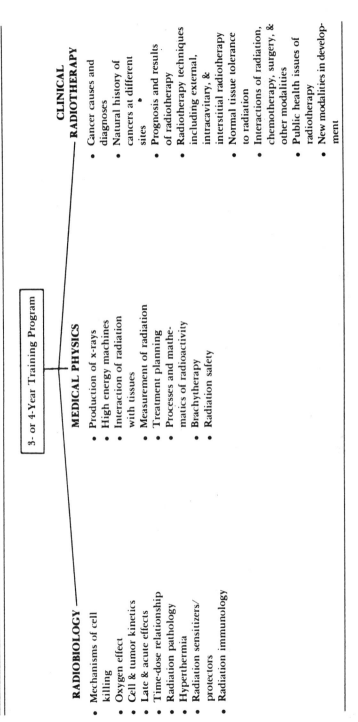

3- or 4-Year Training Program

RADIOBIOLOGY

- Mechanisms of cell killing
- Oxygen effect
- Cell & tumor kinetics
- Late & acute effects
- Time-dose relationship
- Radiation pathology
- Hyperthermia
- Radiation sensitizers/ protectors
- Radiation immunology

MEDICAL PHYSICS

- Production of x-rays
- High energy machines
- Interaction of radiation with tissues
- Measurement of radiation
- Treatment planning
- Processes and mathe- matics of radioactivity
- Brachytherapy
- Radiation safety

CLINICAL RADIOTHERAPY

- Cancer causes and diagnoses
- Natural history of cancers at different sites
- Prognosis and results of radiotherapy
- Radiotherapy techniques including external, intracavitary, & interstitial radiotherapy
- Normal tissue tolerance to radiation
- Interactions of radiation, chemotherapy, surgery, & other modalities
- Public health issues of radiotherapy
- New modalities in develop- ment

failures, or complications arising from such treatments. To deliver good training in medical physics, the department of radiation oncology should be well staffed with physicists not only to handle the day-to-day operation of the department but also to have time for didactic teaching of the residents. The department must also be equipped with various radiotherapy machines so that the residents will be trained to handle various operations of equipment. Usually, only in large departments of radiation oncology do we find a faculty in radiation biology. This person, or his staff, is generally involved heavily in radiation biology research, but a commitment is required also for teaching the residents.

The approach of the radiation oncology department to teaching varies. Some departments emphasize didactic lectures, while others use a seminar structure. Standard text books can often be supplemented with handout pamphlets or syllabi. The American Board of Radiology has set down minimal guidelines for the establishment of a training program in radiation oncology, but the teaching of the psychosocial aspects of radiation oncology is not required.

PSYCHOSOCIAL DEMANDS PLACED ON THE RADIATION ONCOLOGY RESIDENT

The radiation oncology resident is usually the first physician to come in contact with cancer patients when they are referred for radiation treatments. At this point in the patient's disease course, the situation often amounts to emotional crisis, and the referral for radiation treatments engenders a whole new set of fears and questions.

"What is radiation?"

"Is radiation therapy absolutely necessary for me?"

"Is radiation harmful to me?" "What side effects will I have?" "Will I be disabled?" "Will I ever be able to work again?" "Will I ever be able to function as a mother? as a wife? as a husband?"

"Will I become radioactive?" "Will my receiving radiation therapy be harmful to my family?"

Typically, the patient is fearful or angry, and the family, having suffered through multiple diagnostic tests, hospitalization, and, perhaps, surgery, is under enormous stress. Commonly there is a deep-seated fear of the unknown radiation, and of a long course of daily treatments, with real or imagined side effects, of the prognosis, and of the financial/emotional consequences for the loved ones. There may be grief over actual or potential loss (physical, emotional, or financial), leading to depression, active withdrawal from relationships, or isolation engendered by the reactions of family and friends.

The preceding facts are well known and much discussed. What is often not recognized and only rarely spoken of is the emotional reactions of the residents to the patients, the patient's family, and the patient's disease course. Often these reactions and emotions are dealt with in isolation and in a setting of multiple stresses from a variety of sources. Discussions among colleagues are uncommon.

There may be identification with the patient's misfortune. Depending on what the resident's personal past experience is, the illness of an elderly patient, for example, may remind a resident of the illness, suffering, and death of a grandparent. The age, physical appearance, or certain aspects of the medical history may provoke anxiety within the resident about the possibility of his own parents being ill or having cancer. There may be a certain realization of his own mortality, and it is generally acknowledged that the residents have a great sense of sympathy, empathy, and identification with young cancer victims. The resident may have the most difficult time in grappling with acceptance of the reality of the illness of the pediatric cancer patient. The fact that these young patients can potentially have long and useful lives places a great responsibility on the resident who is caring for them.

The patient may be hostile toward physicians. The patient may need to vent his anger at what has befallen him. The resident is often the front-line doctor facing these complex emotions and reactions and may, in the absence of understanding, react with withdrawal or with anger toward the patient or the family.

The resident is taught how to utilize radiation therapy to cure cancer patients. If treatment fails or is attended by significant side effects, the resident may experience guilt. If the resident has developed a bond of friendship with the patient, failure of treatment and often the eventual death of the patient may be accompanied by an overwhelming sense of grief.

The radiation oncology resident is often ill equipped to recognize and handle the emotional stresses that come with caring for cancer patients. Usually young, often fresh out of medical school, and typically not having had much life experience or suffered through a serious illness or loss of a loved one, the resident derives little help from his training. The present day medical school curriculum includes a short rotation through psychiatry, but the emphasis is on an introduction to common psychiatric disorders and nomenclature. Rarely is emphasis placed on recognizing, understanding, and dealing with the psychosocial stresses between ill patients and their physicians. Besides this lack of formal training, the resident often lacks role models. Few of the attending radiation oncologists with whom he works have had such training themselves and can hardly be expected to teach the resident about the psychosocial aspects of radiation oncology. Left to his own devices, the resident may confuse pathological behavior with normal reactions and, with time, may develop a set of maladaptive reactions or coping patterns that will last throughout a professional lifetime.

Clearly, residency training should speak to such issues, but how might this be accomplished? What opportunities might prove useful? Perhaps a clue to one approach might be found in a unique experience in which some of the authors participated at the Mount Zion Hospital.

MOUNT ZION HOSPITAL AND MEDICAL CENTER EXPERIENCE

Between April 1975, and November 1977, Mount Zion Hospital and Medical Center undertook a project, funded by the National Cancer Institute, entitled "Exploratory Studies for Cancer Patients' Rehabilitation." The technique of intensive individual interviews, as well as group discussions, was employed to develop concepts of adaptation and life changes in cancer patients. The results of this study have been reported in detail elsewhere (Castro et al., 1978; Mages et al., 1981).

Sixty adult cancer patients and their families were interviewed extensively in order to analyze their responses to cancer and the factors that correlated with their adaptation to the disease. Two groups of cancer patients were included: patients recently treated and those who were long-term survivors. All of these patients had received radiation therapy as part of their treatments. The acute reactions of patients to their diagnosis and treatment, the possibility of recurrence and progression of disease, the damage to their bodies from illness or from the treatment, and a need to return to a relatively normal life with a sense of self-sufficiency and control were all examined.

Another forty patients and their family members were involved in a discussion group that met weekly for over a year. This format provided them with the opportunity to share experiences and concerns and to explore common problems at length. Two radiation oncology residents were invited to participate in these discussion groups, and each stayed with the group for six months. They were not merely passive observers but played an active role as medical consultants to the group and to the psychiatrist. When questions arose that required clarification regarding medical aspects of radiation treatments, the residents provided this information.

Initially, there were reservations about the presence of a physician at the group meeting. In particular, there were concerns that the participants might be reluctant to express their emotions and feelings. These fears were soon dispelled. The group participants expressed themselves freely, including comments (sometimes negative) about the physicians who had the responsibility for their medical care. The resident rapidly became integrated into the group, interacting with its members and contributing to the discussions.

There were definite advantages to this arrangement, as the resident was able to stay with the group members for six months and therefore came to know the group members quite well, both medically and psychosocially. Outside of the group, there were opportunities for the resident to discuss the various aspects of the group, thereby providing him with an active education, in contrast to a purely passive one consisting of readings, lectures, and the like.

Now, some years later, the residents who participated in this program retain strong impressions of the experience. They feel, without exception, that their exposure to the psychosocial project made them more aware of their patients' needs and more understanding of their emotional turmoil. They feel that this experience had a positive impact on their career development and later clinical practice.

A typical comment was, "I had no idea what the patients were going through until I listened to them. I found out that cancer patients can have different levels of depression. Some patients were obviously sad, while others attempted to put aside their emotions. It became apparent soon that they all had tremendous needs, and I began to appreciate the team approach of emotional support."

Another former resident stated, "I felt that if a physician took the first step to be warm and more attentive in his relationship to his patients, the patients opened up and talked more about their feelings."

They remembered negative feelings as well: "Patients really got on their doctors! Most frequently they were angry and accused their doctors of not telling the truth about their illnesses and their treatments. They were afraid to say these things to the treating physicians, however, for fear that they might jeopardize the relationship and their treatments by doing so. Sometimes the conflicts and the pressures could be quite significant, and the group sessions allowed them to vent their frustrations."

On the subject of training in psychosocial aspects of radiation oncology, one commented, "I feel that formal training will help. We already talked about the importance of residents being in tune with the patients' problems. I feel that it is important for the physician to have more insight about himself as well. Patients 'take out' on the physicians a lot; in other words, unload a lot of their emotions such as anger, anxiety, guilt, etc. The doctor reciprocates by giving up a lot of his 'self' to take care of his patients."

To the question about the influence of the experience with the discussion groups on their career, they answered, "I feel that I have been sympathetic and responsive to my patients, and I am aware that my experience may have contributed to my medical practice. Of course, you can also argue that I participated in the group discussions because I was more inclined to patients' psychological needs in the first place. In any case, I have tended to refer my patients to social workers, psychologists, psychiatrists, or whatever support system there might be."

"I am now working with the local American Cancer Society to recruit clergymen to work together with us. It seems that patients often turn to religion when they have catastrophic illnesses. We have a chaplains' program in our hospital already, a training program for the clergy, and they come to see cancer patients. It will be a great resource for patients' psychosocial support!"

Although it was not the intention of this project to provide training for the radiation oncology residents, it seems that they received a valuable experience from the group discussions. During these sessions, the residents learned about the patients' life stresses, family difficulties, and the patients' images of the radiation oncologist. Complex emotions including anger, doubt, fear, dependence, and so forth came to light. This information was not readily available during the usual patient/doctor encounters such as in treatment rooms, under the therapy machines, or in the examination rooms, where the posture of the meetings was mainly medical and formal. To this day, these previous trainees remain aware of patients' psychosocial needs and tend to refer them to therapy support groups.

PROPOSALS FOR TRAINING PROGRAMS

The experience at Mount Zion Hospital and Medical Center illustrates just one of many possible means by which radiation oncology residents might become more skilled and exposed in various aspects of "psychosocial care of patients." Discussions with the residents who participated in this program revealed other needs of the radiation oncology residents as trainees and as people. "I am often tired and pooped in the evening, and I know that I bring my stresses home. I don't thing that it is good or fair to my family. It would be helpful to recognize the physicians' problems and take care of the doctor as well as the patient. A well-adjusted doctor can take better care of his patients!"

"Doctors are reluctant to talk to each other about personal

feelings and problems. In other words, it is easy to discuss in a remote and objective manner the disease diagnosis, treatment, and management, but it is hard to admit and discuss freely the psychological barriers in patient-doctor relationships. Therefore, it may be that a beneficial environment is needed where problems of the physicians can be talked out."

It is obvious that the first step toward improved training for the radiation oncology resident in the area of psychosocial aspects of cancer must be a recognition by the directors of radiation oncology residency programs of the need to commit time and facilities to provide opportunities for psychosocial training. This is equivalent to nothing more than a commitment to good patient care. A radiation oncology department should not be merely a place where machines are turned on and off but should foster the care of the whole patient.

Formal training in psychosocial aspects of patient care can be given via many avenues, such as rounds, lectures, videotapes, or assigned readings. Skills in counseling should be developed, including recognition of patient needs, whether directly expressed or not. Participation in patient therapy or counseling groups may be very effective. Rotation through a hospice program may offer an enriching experience.

Provision of opportunities for the radiation oncology residents to express their own needs relative to their work is important. This may be in the form of a support group including all the health care providers such as nurses, radiation therapy technicians, other trainees, radiation oncology attending physicians, social workers, and psychologists. The resident, early in training, should be encouraged to verbalize reactions to patients or situations encountered in daily practice.

In summary, the authors believe that there is a real need to understand the psychosocial demands placed on radiation oncology residents and to provide training and experience that will be of use to them personally and to their patients. The authors' perception of the present situation is that such training and experience is virtually nonexistent. They believe firmly that learning to care for the total patient is very important and that this must include the psychosocial aspects as well as the skills of delivering radiation treatments. To remedy the present lack and achieve this objective, directors of residency programs must be made aware of these deficiencies and encouraged to initiate programs to correct them. It is possible that studies funded by appropriate professional groups or governmental agencies may provide a much needed data base and greatly assist in the design of such programs.

REFERENCES

Castro, J.R., N.L. Mages, P. Fobair, G. Mendelsohn, and A. Wolfson. 1978. Final report, Exploratory Studies for Cancer Patient Rehabilitation, to Division of Cancer Research, Resource and Centers and Division of Cancer Control and Rehabilitation, National Cancer Institute, Grant #1 R18 CA16873.

Fiore, N. 1979. Fighting Cancer—One Patient's Perspective. *New England Journal of Medicine, 300* (February):284-89.

Fuller, D.E. 1980. The Transition from Therapeutic Radiologists to Radiation Oncology. *International Journal of Radiation Oncology, Biology, and Physics, 6:*953-54.

Mages, N.L., J.R. Castro, P. Fobair, J.Hall, I. Harrison, G. Mendelsohn, and A. Wolfson. 1981. Patterns of Psychosocial Response to Cancer: Can Effective Adaptation Be Predicted? *International Journal of Radiation Oncology, Biology, and Physics, 7:*385-92.

Peck, A. and J. Boland. 1977. Emotional Reactions to Radiation Treatments, *Cancer, 40:*180-84.

Rosenbaum, E.H. 1975. *Living with Cancer.* New York: Praeger Publishers.

Rosenbaum, E.H., F. Manuel, J. Bray, I.R. Rosenbaum, and A.Z. Cerf. 1978a. *Up and Around: Rehabilitation Exercises for Cancer Patients.* San Francisco: Alchemy Books (Life, Mind, and Body Series).

Rosenbaum, E.H., C.A. Stitt, H. Drasin, I.R. Rosenbaum. 1978b. *Health Through Nutrition: A Comprehensive Guide for the Cancer Patient.* San Francisco: Alchemy Books (Life, Mind and Body Series).

Rotman, M., L. Rogow, G. DeLeon, and N. Heskel. 1977. Supportive Therapy in Radiation Oncology. *Cancer, 39* (suppl): 744-50.

Chapter 16

RADIATION THERAPY RESIDENT
Motivation, Satisfaction, and Implications For the Care of the Cancer Patient

JEROME J. SPUNBERG

R adiation therapy as a medical specialty offers the opportunity to combine close day-to-day patient contact, technical expertise, and stimulating research in a pleasant atmosphere with flexible hours, reasonable income potential, and multiple options for mode of practice. Therefore, it is somewhat surprising that in the United States, with more intense competition for internship and residency positions as a result of an expanding number of graduating medical students, radiation therapy residency programs had, according to 1980 data, remained 28 percent vacant, 42 percent foreign staffed, and largely noncompetitive (*Graduate Medical Education, 1980;* Del Regato and Pittman, 1980).

With these facts in mind, the author undertook to evaluate the factors that have motivated a recent group of residents to enter what he considers to be a highly desirable field, their degree of satisfaction with their selection, their ability and enjoyment in interacting with patients, particularly the terminal patients, and the impact of such contact upon their own lives and attitudes. While the field can be extremely demanding of the psyche, in that ultimate failure is the anticipated outcome in all too many cases, residents may react to these stresses in highly individualistic ways but must maintain composure and present an optimistic and cheerful demeanor to those who turn to them for support.

For those residents properly prepared for and attuned to the needs of the cancer patient, the radiation oncology experience is not only richly rewarding but also a continuing source of personal growth and significance.

THE QUESTIONNAIRES

To evaluate the previously noted factors, questionnaires were mailed to the directors of radiation therapy residencies throughout the United States to be distributed among their trainees. Residency programs generally are three years after previous postgraduate experience or four years without, although some require four years in addition to an internship. Some residents choose to spend one to two years in fellowship immediately upon completion of their residency to increase their knowledge in specific areas such as interstitial implants, newer modalities of radiation, or radiation biology, although the majority enter clinical practice directly. The complete list of ninety-two residencies was obtained from the American Society of Therapeutic Radiologists' directory.

Each questionnaire consisted of forty-five multiple choice or fill in the blank questions. The first third dealt with general information, the middle third with the reasons behind the choice of the field and the residency experience itself, and the last third with patient interactions, attitudes toward death and the dying, the use of religion as a supportive measure, and the existence of cultural, ethnic, or social barriers in relating to patients. An accompanying letter guaranteed anonymity, and only the name of the residency program was specifically requested on a voluntary basis. No attempt was made to gather additional data not provided by the respondents, and there were no subsequent repetitive mailings. Residents were encouraged to complete as much of the questionnaire as they felt they were able and to leave blank one or more questions rather than to discard the whole.

The Results of the Questionnaires

General Results

Of approximately 425 eligible residents or fellows who presumably had access to the questionnaires, 83 responded partially or completely. There were 23 first-year residents, 16 second, 19 third, 16 fourth, and 8 fellows, with one person leaving the item blank. Males outnumbered females 65 to 18, with 61 married, 19 single, 3 divorced, and none widowed. Fifty-two were native-born United States citizens, 9 naturalized United States citizens, and 22 of foreign nationality. Seven of the 22 foreigners were from India, 2 each were from Korea and Great Britain, and no other country had more than one representative. Fifty-five were graduated from American medical schools, and the remaining 28, abroad. The overwhelming majority (62) had already completed at least one year of postgraduate training, in either an internship or a partial or full residency; eighteen had entered radiation therapy residency directly from medical school.

Motivation and the Residency Experience

For both United States citizens and foreigners, patient contact was the major stated reason for entering the field of radiation therapy (Table 16-I). Hours and opportunity were second and third for the group as a whole. Over 50 percent also listed patient contact as the most enjoyable aspect of their work. All respondents felt that patients were benefited by their radiation treatments the majority of the time; no one answered rarely or never. Perhaps as a consequence of this, 73 stated that they would choose the field again, with 6 undecided, 3 unanswered, and only one no. Most

Table 16-I
RESIDENTS' REASONS FOR CHOOSING RT

Reason	1st Choice	2nd Choice	Total
Patient Contact	42	10	52
Hours	11	22	33
Opportunity	11	19	30
Technical	6	13	19
Research	7	8	15
Income Potential	1	0	1
Other	2	2	4
Not Answered	3	9	12
Total	83	83	166

seemed to be enjoying their residency experience and would want to be treated in their own department if they required treatment themselves.

Interactions with Patients

As would be expected, adults over forty comprise the groups treated most frequently in radiation therapy departments, with a large number over sixty. Approximately 50 percent of patients are treated with palliative intent.

Despite the fact that they are only a small fraction of the total patient population, pediatric patients elicited the greatest emotional involvement in almost one-third of the residents who responded to the question. Those closest in age to the residents, the young adult group (ages 21 to 40), were listed most frequently. Residents related best to young and middle-aged adults (Table 16-II).

Approximately 60 percent answered that they were personally affected by the patients they treat less than 25 percent of the time. There was little difference between male and female residents on this point. However, when dealing with terminal patients, 40 of 63 males, or about two-thirds, stated that they were personally affected less than 25 percent of the time, but only 5 of 16 females, or about one-third, said the same (Table 16-III). When the residents of the first two years were compared with those of the last two years or fellowship (Table 16-IV), 24 of 36, or two-thirds, of the former group were personally affected by their terminal

Table 16-II
RELATIONSHIPS OF RESIDENTS WITH PATIENTS BY AGE

Patient Age Group	Treat Most Frequently	Relate to Best	Most Emotionally Involved
Pediatric (under 12)	0	5	22
Adolescent (13-20)	0	2	6
Young Adult (21-40)	0	18	34
Middle-aged Adult (41-60)	52	37	7
Older Adult (over 60)	21	8	6
Not Answered	10	13	8
Total	83	83	83

Table 16-III
PSYCHOLOGICAL EFFECTS ON RESIDENTS OF PATIENT AND TERMINAL
PATIENT CARE VERSUS SEX OF RESIDENT

	% of Patients Affecting Resident Personally					
All Patients	*0-25*	*25-50*	*50-75*	*75-100*	*N.A.*	*Total*
Male Residents	40	12	6	5	2	65
Female Residents	8	5	1	2	2	18
Total	48	17	7	7	4	83
Terminal Patients						
Male Residents	41	10	5	7	2	65
Female Residents	5	7	2	2	2	18
Total	46	17	7	9	4	83

*Not Answered

Table 16-IV
PSYCHOLOGICAL EFFECTS ON RESIDENTS OF TERMINAL PATIENT CARE
VERSUS YEAR OF RESIDENCY

	% of Patients Affecting Resident Personally					
Residency Year	*0-25*	*25-50*	*50-75*	*75-100*	*N.A.*	*Total*
1	11	3	4	4	2	24
2	7	3	2	2	1	15
3	11	4	1	2	1	19
4+	17	6	0	1	0	24
N.A.	0	1	0	0	0	1
Total	46	17	7	9	4	83

*Not Answered

patients less than half the time, as opposed to 38 of 42, or over 90 percent of the more senior residents.

In general, residents were more likely to be involved with terminally ill patients themselves than with their families. Most claimed to be usually or always honest with terminal patients regarding their poor prognosis and rarely avoid answering questions by patients concerning death. As would be expected in a referral specialty, usually radiation therapy residents are not the first physicians to inform the patient with poor prognosis of his chances. Surprisingly, 20 percent answered that they are the first ones more than 50 percent of the time.

Religion is only occasionally encouraged by residents as a supportive measure for their patients. Relationships with clergy were described as worse than those with other physicians, nurses, and social workers, with a larger number leaving that item blank, indicating little contact. The most common religious preference as stated by the residents was Protestant, followed by Jewish, Catholic, and Hindu; fifteen had no religion. Table 16-V shows the relationship between the religious preference of the resident and the use of religion as a supportive measure for patients. Approximately 33 percent (22 of 67) with any religious preference at all rarely or never use it as opposed to 67 percent (10 of 15) of those belonging to no religion.

Finally, only 11 percent of residents usually or frequently experience "cultural, ethnic, or social barriers" in relating to patients. Table 16-VI, however, compares United States citizens to foreigners. Only about 5 percent (3 of 61) of United States citizens usually or frequently encounter such barriers, whereas 25 percent

Table 16-V
USE OF RELIGION AS A SUPPORTIVE MEASURE FOR PATIENTS

Religion of Resident	Use of Religion						
	Always	Usually	Occas.	Rarely	Never	N.A.*	Total
Protestant	0	6	10	4	2	1	23
Jewish	0	4	7	5	0	0	16
Catholic	1	1	5	3	3	0	13
Hindu	0	0	5	2	2	2	11
Moslem	1	1	0	1	0	0	3
Other	0	0	1	0	0	0	1
None	0	2	2	6	4	1	15
Not Answered	0	0	1	0	0	0	1
Total	2	14	31	21	11	4	83

*Not Answered

Table 16-VI
RESIDENTS' NATIONALITY VERSUS CULTURAL, ETHNIC, OR SOCIAL
BARRIERS IN RELATING TO PATIENTS

Nationality of Resident	Barriers in Relating to Patients						
	Usually	Freq.	Occas.	Rarely	Never	N.A.*	Total
U.S.A.							
native	0	3	21	26	2	0	52
naturalized	0	0	1	5	2	1	9
Foreign citizen	1	5	5	6	3	2	22
Total	1	8	27	37	7	3	83

*Not Answered

(6 of 22) of residents of foreign nationality do. The naturalized citizen group is too small to be dealt with specifically.

DISCUSSION

It is not likely that the questionnaire respondents represent a true sampling of the radiation therapy resident group as a whole. Since only 28 of the 83 residents were foreign medical graduates (34%), as compared to approximately 50 percent of all residents in the field in the United States, the views of American medical graduates are overrepresented in these data. The reasons for this are unclear but may relate to decreased access to the questionnaires, difficulty in understanding the questions, fear of expressing their opinions, or a negative attitude toward the questionnaire itself so as to place it at a lower priority compared to other tasks.

The respondents most probably comprise the more highly motivated or opinionated minority of the residency group regarding the field or the psychosocial aspects of cancer patient care. It is apparent that the overwhelming majority are quite satisfied with their work, feel that they usually benefit their patients with radiation therapy, and would make the same career choice given the opportunity. In addition, patient contact was the motivating factor behind their choice and is the aspect that they enjoy most in their day-to-day routine. Some of the other advantages of the field such as hours, opportunity, and technical considerations also contributed to the decision, but income potential played a lesser role.

As expected, most patients treated in radiation therapy departments are over forty years old with many over sixty, and about half are treated for palliation and half for cure. It is of interest that residents were more often emotionally involved with the under-forty group of patients and particularly the pediatric group, whom they treat far more infrequently. This is consistent with the fact that 60 percent responded that they rarely are personally affected by their patients as a whole, since so many are in the older age categories. Terminal patients did not appear to elicit a different response compared to all patients, although female residents and more junior residents were more likely to become emotionally involved with the terminally ill than male or senior residents.

It is surprising and somewhat disturbing that 20 percent responded that they are the first physicians to inform the patient with poor prognosis of his chances. There must be many patients who come for treatment not knowing the nature of their disease and its outcome and some who are completely misinformed either intentionally or unintentionally. This conclusion is well known to most radiation therapists, who frequently discover the "bad news" has been left to them to tell. Since almost all the residents stated that they are generally honest with terminal patients regarding their prognosis, it is apparent that when the patient asks, he will be told, and perhaps many do not ask until the time comes when they must sign an informed consent requiring adequate preliminary preparation.

Once patients are aware of their situation, or even while they merely suspect, they often turn to residents for emotional support. Residents as a rule are more accessible and have more routine contact with their patients in radiation therapy departments for treatment field corrections, prescriptions for side effects, or follow-up of response during the treatment course than attending physicians. Only 11 percent of the residents admitted frequent cultural, ethnic, or social barriers in relating to patients, with a higher percentage among the residents of foreign nationality. This may be due to language problems in some cases but to more deeply rooted cultural differences in others. The number may be higher among those who did not respond to the questionnaire. As evidenced by their use of religion, residents tend to project their own beliefs and attitudes upon their patients. Those belonging to no religion rarely or never use it two-thirds of the time as a supportive measure for patients as compared to one-third of the time for those with any religion at all. Since it is highly unlikely that residents with a religious preference treat patients with religious views significantly differently from residents with no religion, the use of religion depends primarily upon the resident, not the patient. This is not in the best interest of the patient, as deep religious conviction may provide solace or security in the face of serious illness, an emotional resource not as available to the patient whose doctor lacks religious affiliation. The physician usually must tap every potential source of strength in dealing with the cancer patient, especially the terminal patient.

CONCLUSION

The results of the questionnaires reveal a fairly distinct group of residents who selected the field of radiation therapy during medical school or other postgraduate training and by and large are enjoying their residency experience and interactions with patients. Most entered the field for patient contact and derive the greatest satisfaction from this aspect of their training despite their diverse backgrounds. It would seem that the problem in attracting qualified candidates to the discipline is one of introduction rather than persuasion. Greater and earlier contact with radiation therapists and their patients, with concomitant dissolution of misconceptions and fears, would undoubtedly fill the vacant residency positions with numbers to spare. As the availability of positions for well-trained radiation therapists dwindles each year despite the shortage of residents, perhaps it is the good fortune of those currently in residency that the "word has not gotten out."

REFERENCES

Del Regato, J.A. and D.D. Pittman. 1980. The Training of Radiotherapists in the United States. *International Journal of Radiation Oncology, Biology and Physics, 6:*1705-10.

Graduate Medical Education in the United States. 1980. *Journal of the American Medical Association, 243:*867-87.

Chapter 17

THE RADIATION THERAPY TECHNOLOGIST

PATRICIA CHAMBERS

he competent physician, before he attempts to give medicine to his patients, makes himself acquainted not only with the disease which he wishes to cure, but also with the habits and constitution of the sick man." This statement, made by Cicero in *DeOratori II* over 2,000 years ago, demonstrates that although the physician's primary role is to cure the disease, he must be concerned with the whole person and not just the disease. The physician was named by Cicero as the caregiver. Advances in medical knowledge have required the expansion of the caregiver concept to include a caregiving team, of which the technologist is an integral part. In the past some physicians have tried to minimize the importance of the technologist. This is no longer possible. The exacting requirements of today's treatments place an increasing burden on all members of the radiation therapy team. Each member has gained expertise in his area, and the cooperation among them produces the maximum benefit for the patient.

As an educator, the author has often been asked to describe the difference between radiation therapy, diagnostic radiology, and nuclear medicine. Having worked in all three, the author feels the technical demands to be the same; however, the difference occurs with the technologist's relationship to the patient. In the latter two disciplines, the technologist sees the patient once or infrequently. The meeting is usually impersonal, even though the technologist is friendly and caring; the transient nature of the meeting makes it impersonal. The radiation therapy technologist sees the patient daily for several weeks, and the nature of the meeting and the subsequent relationship is different for both patient and technologist. The patient places his trust in the technologist, as he has in the physician. Since technologists see patients daily and physicians usually do not, the technologist acts as a liaison between the two. The technologist has a great responsibility toward the patient and must be caring and empathetic without becoming personally involved. This is often difficult and sometimes impossible. The bond formed between the technologist and patient is, in the author's opinion, the major difference between this specialty and others.

The role of the technologist varies with the institution, and it is difficult to assess the degree of, and difference in, responsibility among hospital departments. In major teaching hospitals, the presence of a resident staff influences the types and amounts of responsibility. On the other hand, when working in a private office or community hospital, the technologist's responsibilities, in addition to the standard duties, may include treatment planning, nursing, and social work.

All members of the radiation therapy team are special. Technologists give a great deal to their patients. They see an average of twenty to forty patients every day. They must be able to boost egos and lick wounds, to encourage certain patients to eat and discourage others from drinking, to talk to families and social workers, to arrange appointment times, and—one of the most difficult tasks—explain to the patients why they must wait for their treatment.

Many of the patients are in pain. Although radiation therapy is a primary method of treatment for controlling pain from bony metastasis, too frequently it is not effective on patients. Treating them daily, placing them in uncomfortable positions, and trying to reassure them the pain will disappear can be emotionally draining.

Technologists may treat children as part of their routine duties. Although they are usually cooperative, one cannot help considering the outrage of a child with malignant disease.

Because of the nature of the disease, radiotherapy patients are terrified of dying. They exhibit this fear in many ways. Some become hostile, others euphoric, and still others very quiet. Some patients are hyperalert, and the technologist must be constantly aware that an innocent remark may be misinterpreted.

Due to the patient's real or imagined limited life span, time is one of the few things he wants to control. In radiation therapy, time is at a premium. Technologists are constantly torn between setting up the new, sometimes unscheduled patient and treating their regular patients. Fitting another patient into an already full treatment schedule is difficult for all involved. Every technologist has felt at times as if he were working on an assembly line. The ability to work rapidly must be developed to move the patient through treatment as quickly as possible without appearing rushed or uncaring.

Patients often ask very pointed questions about the nature of their illnesses. Although it is not the technologist's job to confirm or deny the presence of malignant disease, ignoring the questions is not a solution either. Much has been written on the subject of patients' awareness of the diagnosis. Frequently, the physician, family, and/or patient are involved in the denial. All three are aware of the patient's prognosis, yet none can discuss it openly. Technologists are often caught in the middle of this war of minds, and patients may choose them, the neutral observers, to discuss their illness or impending death. Should they encourage their desire to talk or discourage them by saying it is all nonsense and risk losing their confidence? Should they neglect to reassure patients for fear of lying to or misleading them, or is this acting on their own conscious or unconscious fear of death?

The questions and problems of working in this profession are real, and the answers elusive. Dr. Lothar Gidro-Frank (n.d.), a psychiatrist who studied technologists during their normal routine, made the following observations:

> Radiotherapy technologists have little freedom and no opportunity to work independently, creatively and at their own pace. Day after day they are tied to the machines they operate as well as the schedule set up for them. Pressure is increased when they are forced to treat unscheduled patients on an attending's say so.
>
> Residents and attendings wander around, usually ready to correct, at times to criticize, seldom to praise. Set-ups and lengths of treatment are often changed, and the technologist has to bear the brunt of the

patient's resultant anxiety, anger or depression. The pressure to treat patients fast yet accurately weighs heavily on the technologist's shoulder.

Technologists find it a burden to face patients with severe pain, depression, or manifestly incurable illness. The "assembly line" aspect of the work does not permit sufficient interaction between patients and staff and is discouraging.

Some technologists are valued for their speed in setting up and getting a patient in and out, others for their deliberate precision, again others for being especially understanding with patients, and still others because they are good with children. Different staff members rate others somewhat inconsistently. What is most often overlooked in evaluating a technologist's work is the kindness with which he or she treats the patients. They are the patient's conduit to the doctor. Above all, they sustain hope, which is the mainstay of life.

In a paper entitled "Cancer Patients' Evaluations of Radiation Therapy Services" by Larry Smith (1980), the author briefly assesses the relationship between the patient and technologist. Mr. Smith reports that 100 percent rated their relationship as either good or excellent, 42 percent reported the technologists were friendly, and 58 percent said they were warm and caring. All the comments about the technologists were favorable and indicate how important they are in the treatment process, especially in establishing meaningful relationships with the patient.

The technical demands of the job are well known; however, the psychological demands are difficult to evaluate. Just as patients exhibit numerous mechanisms of coping with their disease, technologists must find various ways of defending themselves from the emotional demands of the job. Certain technologists prefer to remain ignorant of the patient's history and rarely ask about their progress when they return for checkups. Other staff members create an emotional distance by placing a barrier between themselves and the patient. Early in their careers technologists learn to detach themselves emotionally and leave their patients at work. Once in a while, however, a patient will "get to them," and that patient's daily treatment becomes an emotional chore.

Smith's paper indicates that "staff members need to acknowledge the impact working with seriously ill patients can have on their professional and personal lives. Support and counseling services should also be made available to staff members" (Smith, 1980). While emotional and psychological support may be provided for the patient, it is rarely available for the staff. Gidro-Frank, as part of his study of radiation therapy departments, organized the members of the staff into a group for just this purpose. The results were mixed. Attendance was erratic, and most were unwilling or unable to open up. Some progress was made on certain issues of mutual concern. In the author's opinion, the result of the group experience would have been unequivocal if it were conducted in another department with a different working atmosphere. The author personally benefited greatly from the experience. It enabled her to understand the patients' actions and her reactions to them. It made many aspects of the job easier. It was also helpful just to have a discussion in which one could "get things off your chest." Any assistance in enabling technologists to maintain that delicate balance between making themselves available for as much support as humanly possible without succumbing to emotions that destroy their equanimity and interfere with their performance is appreciated.

What made technologists choose this particular profession? For some physicians and technologists it was the attractiveness of the working conditions, no evenings and weekends. Others chose the profession because a close relative or friend was hospitalized or had received radiation therapy. Others entered the field with very little knowledge of the demands of the profession. Whatever the reasons, which are numerous, the profession seems to be populated with technically capable, caring individuals who can foster better relationships among staff members.

In selecting students, the future technologists, educators should acquaint them with the demands of the profession, both technical and emotional. It is unfair to the student and the profession to educate individuals whose primary motivation for choosing radiation therapy is the availability of jobs.

Technologists are often asked, "How can you work in that field? What are the rewards?" Particularly gratifying is the child who returns for a checkup five years posttreatment for Wilm's tumor or the young woman, treated for Hodgkin's disease, who returns for her annual checkup with her recently born son. The gratitude in the eyes of patients and family and the thanks expressed in so many ways make up for any depressing moments.

REFERENCES

Gidro-Frank, L. n.d. In-service Education Lecture. Columbia-Presbyterian Medical Center, New York, New York.

Smith, L. 1980. Cancer Patients' Evaluations of Radiation Therapy Services. *Radiologic Technology, 51(5):*601-609.

THE ISSUE OF SHARED RESPONSIBILITY

EDWARD H. GILBERT

I start writing about the topic of the physician's sharing responsibility with the patient with my own fatigue apparent. Over the past five years, I have manifested great enthusiasm on this subject at times. Now I am tired. Although I have seen a few people be brave and show courage that would make any of us glow with appreciation for the human spirit, I have seen many more suffer, stopping their lives long before breathing ceased, long before cancer symptoms had manifested themselves.

I pleaded with some to change parts of their lives, I observed and empathized with others, and I was a technician entering the path of many. The common threads of the meaning of life, the root of our essence, and the nature of our spirit were woven through all the life histories studied and are the basis for this chapter. Unlike most medical papers, this report will be told from the heart as well as the intellect. This is a tale of two characters, the healer and the person being healed. It will not always be clear which is the physician and which is the patient.

In the past the training of the physician directly reflected the priorities set by society. Technical expertise was praised throughout the training period. The effect of the rigid schedule on the physician's life was not addressed. There were hours of study to learn this important information, but a sacrifice was made. Rarely did a balance exist in the personal lives. Personal development and experience in the humanities were at times overlooked. In retrospect, there did not appear to be any choice.

The alternative, academic failure, was unacceptable. As a person, the physician by his very training method could be years behind in social evolution, yet society considered his medical degree to be the equivalent of a doctorate in all of life's activities (sex, religion, psychology, spirituality). With this background and training, he faced the critical challenge of suddenly becoming the total physician, expert in cancer and all its social ramifications. In order to control his own environment and the feelings of insecurity that were beyond his technical expertise, some definition of his role became mandatory. Frequently, an authoritarian role fit most comfortably.

The mysterious nature of malignant diseases and the patient's loss of physical control when such a diagnosis is made cause feelings of helplessness in many. The meeting of physician and patient offers a perfect opportunity for the patient to relinquish his last remnant of control. Social expectations support giving power to the physician, leaving responsibility for the cure in the hands of the person who "knows all." In the past, many physicians supported this response further by desiring total authority, making it easier to apply the technical aspects of the usually morbid treatment without anxiety-producing controversy. Health care was a one-way street—physician to patient—with active authority from the physician and passive acceptance by the sick person.

In the past ten to fifteen years, the sciences of psychosomatic medicine, mind-body interaction, and self-responsibility for health have gained credibility. This new knowledge has caused a schism in roles. There is now a question of who is ultimately responsible for health and disease. A new dimension has been added to the armamentarium for health and/or recovery from disease—the patient's own motivation. Education can influence the patient's emotional and psychological state, his stress level, and his nutritional state and physical exercise status. The patient can now meet the physician without relinquishing personal responsibility. Yet, even most who are knowledgeable are not willing to take this stand. Frequently, in the mind of the patient, the doctor alone stands at the crossroads of life and death, and his decisions direct the path ultimately taken. However, both can walk the road together if the reality of both partners is in agreement. The creation of this synergism is the challenge.

In 1976, the Cancer Self-Help Program was started at Presbyterian Medical Center (Denver, Colorado) to teach cancer patients the tools for personal health and self-responsibility. It was partially based on the work of Carl and Stephanie Simonton (Simonton et al., 1978) and had many phases. For the initial year, it was eight weeks in length, and fifty patients participated. For the next three years a shortened twenty-four hour, two weeks in length program was conducted every three months for ten to twenty patients, each with a family member. About 200 patients took this course. Finally, twelve patients who had completed the initial course entered a thirteen-week intensive advanced program. A general overview of the content will be presented, with the overall result being improved quality of life and quality of death for most of those involved. The essence of what happened to the patients can be described. There is no way to tell each story; however, it must be stressed that each person did have an individual path. This collective report is an attempt to organize their individual experiences.

As long as a person is feeling emotional chaos, nothing constructive can be accomplished psychologically. The issues surrounding the diagnosis of cancer must be clarified in regard to prognosis, appropriate treatment, and side effects of the therapy or as a result of the cancer process itself. Until this is accomplished, most people will be oriented toward survival problems. Acute intervention resources are very valuable and allow for more rapid movement through this difficult initial period. Volunteer organizations staffed by previously treated cancer patients, social workers, nurses, technicians, friends, and family members can provide important input. Once the survival issues are clarified, most individuals find that they have a unique opportunity. They can restructure their priorities and receive peer and social acceptance for their decisions since they are in a life-threatening situation. Unfortunately, very few people take advantage of this opportunity.

Those who do and are willing to go further into personal exploration usually accept the belief that life events, positive as well as negative, have meaning within the context of their personal growth. To imply that getting a disease such as cancer has life meaning connotes an attached responsibility for the eventual emotional outcome of the process. It is recognized that personal belief systems and attitudes are under a person's control, but it is very difficult to believe that one can learn from one's disease. Guilt for not making appropriate changes, for feeling anxiety and resentment, and for having too much stress in life are negative psychological mechanisms that can be the side effects of taking the stance of personal responsibility. Therefore, our program dealt with these issues first, teaching that these responses are natural and can be put in perspective.

Stress in our lives, difficult life situations, unhappiness, and feelings of being trapped by the environment are common life events to some degree. There is an attempt to make things better by making proper decisions, but more often than not the options available for solving the problems are unknown. This is reflected in the following story from Alan Wheeler:

> I open the door of my car, sit behind the wheel, and notice in the corner of vision an ant scurrying about on the smooth barren surface of the concrete parking lot, doomed momentarily to be crushed by one of the thousand passing wheels. There exists, however, a brilliant alternative for this gravely endangered creature; in a few moments a woman will appear with a picnic basket and we shall drive to the sunny hilltop meadow. This desperate ant has but to climb the wheel of my car to a safe sheltered ledge, and in half an hour will be in a paradise for ants. But this option, unknown, unknowable, yields no freedom to the ant, who is doomed, and the only irony belongs to me who observes, who reflects on the options potentially as meaningful to me that may be eluding my awareness at the moment as this option is to the ant.

What we know we know, and what we do not know we do not know. However, we can educate ourselves to new options, giving ourselves better choices for future decisions. A poor decision made in the past was the best we could do with the knowledge we had at the time, and holding on to guilt about that life event is draining and nonconstructive. Teaching people these concepts over six to eight hours of group work and counseling sets a foundation for emotional growth and learning from the disease.

Clarity leads to solutions. The nature of consciousness is to be able to solve problems only after they are recognized. For people with disease, this means reflection on their lives at the time of the onset of their disease. They need to recall life events, attach meaning and significance to stressful and uncomfortable times, and, in contrast, recognize happy periods. The clarity that reflection brings allows priorities to be set. Having people write down the stresses in their lives can be a powerful experience. The physical act of writing these thoughts creates substance and adds reality to fleeting ideas. To be able to interpret negative life experiences without feelings of guilt and regret can be a major turning point on the path to self-understanding.

Patients' views of their identity and self-worth were interwoven throughout their perception of previous life events. Much like society in general, it was certainly not unique to find the patients in the program concerned about their self-esteem. However, these people with cancer seemed to have lower feelings of self-esteem than the rest of society, but this could have been related to having a disease such as cancer. Loss of self-respect, loss of control over bodily functions, and loss of job security were all reasons for losing self-esteem. New psychological techniques taught principles that helped people to recognize special qualities within themselves, thereby boosting feelings of self-worth.

Using biofeedback to teach patients how to influence their physiology was another tool utilized in the program. As mentioned previously, many people saw their cancer as loss of control over their body's physiology. Teaching people to influence autonomic nervous system function, such as extremity temperature, sweating response, muscle contractions, and brain waves provided experiential learning about self-regulation of the body. Suddenly, the body was not totally dissociated from conscious influence. This regaining of some measure of control seemed to eliminate part of the fear associated with the disease process. Patients could now contribute to their treatment in a positive way by reducing stress levels and decreasing side effects such as nausea and pain. In conjunction with biofeedback, instruction in meditation and visual imagery provided tools for active participation in treatment. Picturing pleasant environments and positive disease outcomes, plus focusing on goals of future desired life events, helped the patient's attitude. It was important to teach these specific tools, since the positive emotions they create were quickly apparent and reinforced the desire to share responsibility.

An important crossroad in the program revolved around secondary gains of disease. Patients did not like the thought that they gained something by being sick. Yet, acceptance that benefit can come from difficult life situations was important. Identifying the particular advantage of being ill, i.e. time off from work, attention from the family, the ability to say no, gave impetus to concentrating on methods of achieving the same goal while healthy. The technique was to focus on life situations that change for the better only while illness is present and then to mold these priorities into life situations that are present with health.

Goals and purpose in life are complex subjects. One can talk about fun and recreational goals, job-related goals, and personal growth goals. Yet, there is a deeper subject involving a perceived reason for being (a purpose for life). In their search many people come upon unique and creative reasons for living. More often than not, the orientation is toward external purposes for living (family, job), but some look within to find meaning. The form this meaning takes is related to each person's feeling of internal destiny, the intuition of one's own path. Pursuit of internal growth, of feeling, of being needed, of moving in some direction, is part of this evolutionary process. The common thread seems to be the internal searching for a reason for life. The paths are many, but they all lead to this central theme. Our program explored this subject and helped many to come closer to their own truths.

Internal awareness, decreased suffering by attaching meaning to the suffering, and personal growth from the disease process were the essence of the program. With the insights obtained, many patients could create a totally new and different perspective about the disease. One can imagine the communication problems these people had with physicians. Most physicians have never faced these in their own lives, so to expect them to understand the patient's experience was unfair. Yet, the patient desired an orientation of shared responsibility, and there was disappointment when the doctor did not desire or understand this. Communication gaps were created, causing anxiety for both patient and physician. Complaints about the physician's "not listening" were made, but one must remember that this did not represent a change from previous behavior on the physician's part. It was just new recognition by the patient that he had chosen a new role. For the doctor, listening to an idea that one does not wish to apply in one's own life is threatening, so the hearing stops. For shared responsibility to be effective, both partners must be part of the process and be able to apply it to their own lives. Today, many physicians are part of this evolutionary change, thus the potential for synergism exists more now than at any previous time.

I have described a program that 250 patients were part of over a period of four years. I am a radiation therapist and participated in the care of thousands of cancer patients in the same time period. Those patients who overlapped my radiation practice and the Self-Help Program were the ones who taught me about shared responsibility. But, in trying to relate to my other patients over the years, gaps became apparent. Interactions were superficial and disease oriented. These patients were not interested in self-help. For me, this was disappointing, since I knew that with motivation these people could do more to contribute to their recovery. I realized the hard way that you cannot make people do things for themselves and that this approach is not appropriate for everyone. My interactions with patients were on many levels, acting with some as coparticipant in the process and with many more as technical director of their treatment.

I started this chapter by saying that it might be difficult to separate what applies to the patient from what is oriented to the physician. I felt as if I were on both roads, learning tools and evolving my inner growth along with the patients. I was their teacher, and they were mine. At times the line of distinction between healer and healee merged. Shared responsibility was, in actuality, sharing life and its events. These moments were revitalizing for me. Furthermore, responsibility for the outcome was not mine alone. I had more to offer than just technical expertise and was effective in ways that the phrase "being a healer for the body, mind, and spirit" connotes. I was listened to, and I listened. I advised and took advice. I taught and was taught. I shared in another's life and felt respect for my role as a physician.

I am tired but not discouraged. Our society is beginning to appreciate the importance of the individual and his search for inner meaning. More people are utilizing negative life events as times for change and learning. More are respecting the vitality of their life and spirit. With these changes a new paradigm of health is emerging. It speaks of embracing disease as a friend and teacher, as a time for reflection and change, and as an opportunity to regain health so that the inner destiny of humans can be completed for their lifetime. With this path, the time near death is a time when it is known that a full lifetime has been lived, however long.

REFERENCES

Simonton, O.C., S. Matthews-Simonton, and J. Creighton. 1978. *Getting Well Again.* Los Angeles: J.P. Tarcher.

Chapter 19

THE ROLE OF THE RADIOBIOLOGIST IN RADIATION ONCOLOGY

Kenneth L. Mossman

T he successful management of the cancer patient by radiation involves the integrated efforts of a number of medical and allied medical specialties including radiation oncology, radiation physics, radiation therapy technology, nursing, social work, and radiobiology. Figure 19-1 illustrates how these various disciplines may interact in a radiation oncology department.

There are two major objectives in the radiation management of the cancer patient: (a) to rid the patient of his disease and (b) to minimize injury to the surrounding normal tissues. Except for radiobiology, all disciplines shown in Figure 19-1 are involved directly in the care of the patient in order to achieve these objectives.

Even though the radiobiologist is not involved directly in patient care, he can play an important role in radiation oncology by applying himself to the clinical problems of the oncologist and by providing instruction to the oncologist and supporting staff in the biological principles of radiation oncology. The purpose of this chapter is to describe the role of the radiobiologist in a radiation oncology setting and the ways he may contribute to patient care.

J. Robert Andrews, M.D., provided valuable advice in the preparation of this chapter. Part of this work was supported by a grant from the National Institutes of Health, National Cancer Institute (CA-18865).

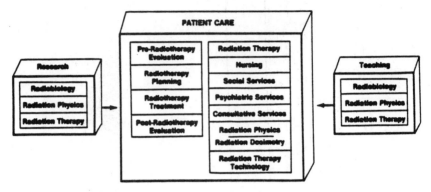

Figure 19-1. The effective management of the cancer patient by radiation involves complex cooperation among a number of disciplines, including those listed under patient care. These disciplines are associated to varying degrees in pre- and postradiotherapy evaluation and radiotherapy planning and treatment. Research and teaching, especially in radiation biology, physics, and therapy, are important activities that influence patient care in a radiation oncology department.

DEFINITION OF RADIOBIOLOGY

Radiobiology is a basic science of radiation oncology and is concerned with the biological effects of radiation exposure. In the context of radiation oncology, radiobiology is specifically concerned with the effects of ionizing radiations on neoplastic normal cells and tissues and in developing and implementing methods to increase the radiosensitivity of tumors and decrease the sensitivity of normal tissues. Radiobiology is an interdisciplinary field encompassing various aspects of physics, chemistry, mathematics, and biology; training in radiobiology usually demands extensive graduate work in some or all of these disciplines.

Activities of a radiobiologist in a radiation oncology department include teaching, participation in clinical conferences, and research (Table 19-I).

TEACHING

The education of the radiation oncologist and the supporting staff concerning the biological principles of radiotherapy is an important role of the radiobiologist. A clear understanding of the

Table 19-I
ROLE OF THE RADIOBIOLOGIST IN RADIATION ONCOLOGY

Teaching
    Radiation oncologist and supporting staff
    Medical students and residents

Participation in Clinical Conferences

Research
    Design of clinical trials
    Development of radioprotective and radiosensitizing compounds
    Evaluation of normal and neoplastic tissue response
    Evaluation of new radiation modalities and combined modalities

underlying biological mechanisms and phenomena in radiotherapy is an important adjunct in the care of the cancer patient. For instance, if the social worker, nutritionist, and psychologist have a basic understanding of the biological basis of radiotherapy, then more effective care strategies may be developed by them. General topics usually covered in radiobiology lectures may vary widely. Some topic outlines have been previously published (Baker, 1975; Howland et al., 1976). Radiobiology is also an integral part of the radiology and radiation oncology resident teaching program and may be taught as part of an overall introduction to oncology to medical students. Exposure to the principles of radiobiology early in a medical student's training may be useful not only to develop an understanding of radiation oncology but also to develop an appreciation for the uses and hazards of radiation in medicine.

CLINICAL CONFERENCES

The radiobiologist should be encouraged to attend clinical conferences. These conferences provide the radiobiologist with the opportunity to discuss various clinical problems with respect to radiobiological mechanisms. In this way the relevance of radiobiology to radiation oncology may be emphasized (Baker, 1975).

RESEARCH

Radiation biology can continue to make significant contributions to the practice of radiotherapy through research efforts in the laboratory and clinic. By applying himself to the clinical problems of the radiation oncologist, the radiobiologist can influence the practice of radiation oncology (Lindop, 1973). The radiobiologist can provide input into the design, conduct, and interpretation of clinical trials in which new treatment techniques, modalities, or radiation response modifiers are being investigated. Radiobiologists have made significant contributions to the development and clinical implementation of radioprotective compounds such as WR-2721 and hypoxic cell radiosensitizers (Denekamp, 1980; Kligerman et al., 1980).

Significant developments have been made by radiobiologists in the development and implementation of high linear energy transfer (LET) radiations (Hall, 1976) and in the combined uses of radiation and chemotherapeutic agents in the treatment of neoplastic diseases.

Of critical importance to the effective use of radiation in the treatment of cancer is the knowledge of normal and neoplastic tissue responses to radiation. With this information, the radiation oncologist can properly adjust dosage and treatment portals to maximize effects to the tumor while causing minimal damage to surrounding critical normal tissues. For the management of many tumors, the effects of radiation on the surrounding normal tissues are often dose limiting and must be considered an integral part of the therapy from the viewpoint of morbidity (Mossman and Scheer, 1977). Normal tissue response in the radiotherapy of head and neck tumors is a good case in point. Damage to the salivary glands and gustatory tissues is an especially serious problem resulting in or contributing to dry mouth, taste loss, mucositis, rampant tooth decay, and difficulties in the maintenance of adequate nutrition. The temporal development and severity of these complications are not well understood by radiation oncologists and represent an area where the radiobiologist can make a contribution.

Radiobiologists have studied salivary dysfunction and taste loss in patients given radiotherapy to the head and neck (Mossman and Henkin, 1978; Mossman et al., 1981). In salivary function studies a 50 percent decrease in parotid salivary flow and a 60 percent decrease in parotid salivary protein after one week of therapy were observed. This salivary dysfunction continued during therapy. Measured taste loss data in eighteen patients prior to and immediately after therapy are shown (Table 19-II). Prior to therapy, patients had measurable taste loss. Thresholds were 80 percent higher in these patients as compared to thresholds in normal volunteers (see Table 19-II). In fact, over 90 percent of head and neck cancer patients have measurable taste loss prior to any therapy (Mossman and Henkin, 1978). After therapy, taste loss increased dramatically such that thresholds were four times higher than normal (see Table 19-II). Measurements of taste loss and salivary dysfunction in patients one to seven years after therapy indicate that these complications may persist in some patients long after the completion of treatment (Mossman et al., 1982).

Patients not only have measurable changes in taste and salivary function but also complain of loss of taste, abnormal taste sensations, anorexia, and dry mouth. Frequencies of these subjective complaints before and after radiotherapy are shown in Table 19-II. Significant increases in the frequency of these subjective complaints were noted after therapy was completed. In addition, patients are frequently in pain and have difficulty swallowing and eating because of the oral tissue damage resulting from curative courses of radiotherapy (Chencharick and Mossman, 1983).

The management of these complications illustrates the importance of a multidisciplinary approach for the care of a patient. The studies reported here indicate the varied and complex signs and symptoms associated with the complications of the radiotherapy of head and neck cancer. Clearly, the radiation oncologist and the nutritionist, social worker, nurse, dentist, and other members of the radiation oncology support staff can play a significant role in alleviating these problems during and after therapy. The radiobiologist may play an important role by assisting the radiation oncologist in defining the nature and severity of complications in quantitative terms as well as by developing preventive measures.

CONCLUSION

Radiobiology can significantly contribute to radiation oncology by providing educational and research services and by participa-

Table 19-II
TASTE LOSS AND SUBJECTIVE COMPLAINTS IN RADIOTHERAPY PATIENTS

| | Measured Taste Loss* | Subjective Complaints | | | |
		Taste Loss	Abnormal Taste Sensations	Anorexia	Dry Mouth
Prior to Radiotherapy	1.8	1/18‡	2/18	3/18	2/18
After Radiotherapy†	4.0	12/18	12/18	9/18	12/18

*Taste loss is defined as the ratio of taste thresholds in patients to thresholds in normal volunteers. Numbers are the geometric means of ratios for detection and recognition thresholds for salt, sweet, sour, and bitter qualities.

†All patients (N=18) had tumors of the head and neck and were treated with a Co-60 teletherapy source using conventional treatment techniques. Total radiation doses ranged from 60-66 gray (6,000-6,600 rad) given in 6½ to 8 weeks. Details of patient population have been published elsewhere (Mossman and Henkin, 1978).

‡Fraction of patients with subjective complaint.

tion in clinical conferences. However, the effectiveness and usefulness of the radiobiologist can only be realized if there is appropriate support and cooperation from other members of the radiation oncology department.

REFERENCES

Baker, D. 1975. Radiobiology and the Role of the Radiobiologist in the Context of a Teaching-oriented Radiation Oncology Department. *Radiologia Clinic, 44:*579-86.

Chencharick, J. and K. Mossman. 1983. Nutritional Consequences of the Radiotherapy of Head and Neck Cancer. *Cancer, 51:*811-15.

Denekamp, J. 1980. Testing of Hypoxic Cell Radiosensitizers *in Vivo. Cancer Clinical Trials, 3:*139-48.

Hall, E. 1976. Radiation and the Single Cell: The Physicist's Contribution to Radiobiology. *Physics in Medicine and Biology, 21:*347-59.

Howland, W., M. Baker, D. Pizzarello, E. Hall, M. Schreiber, R. Schulz, D. Starchman, and R. Tanner. 1976. RSNA Syllabus for Radiation Biology in Diagnostic Radiology Resident Training. *Radiology, 120:*233-36.

Kligerman, M., M. Shaw, M. Slavid, and J. Yuhas. 1980. Phase I Clinical Studies with WR 2721. *Cancer Clinical Trials, 3:*217-21.

Lindop, P. 1973. Radiotherapy, Radiobiology—Can Radiobiology Contribute? *British Journal of Radiology, 46:*799-802.

Mossman, K. and R. Henkin. 1978. Radiation-induced Changes in Taste Acuity in Cancer Patients. *International Journal of Radiation Oncology, Biology and Physics, 4:*663-70.

Mossman, K. and A. Scheer. 1977. Complications of the Radiotherapy of Head and Neck Cancer. *Ear, Nose, and Throat Journal, 56:*145-49.

Mossman, K., A. Shatzman, and J. Chencharick. 1981. Effects of Radiotherapy on Human Parotid Saliva. *Radiation Research, 88:*403-12.

Mossman, K., A. Shatzman, and J. Chencharick. 1982. Long-term Effects of Radiotherapy on Taste and Salivary Function in Man. *International Journal of Radiation Oncology, Biology and Physics, 8:*991-97.

INDEX